THE INSPIRED APRON

A Recipe for Life

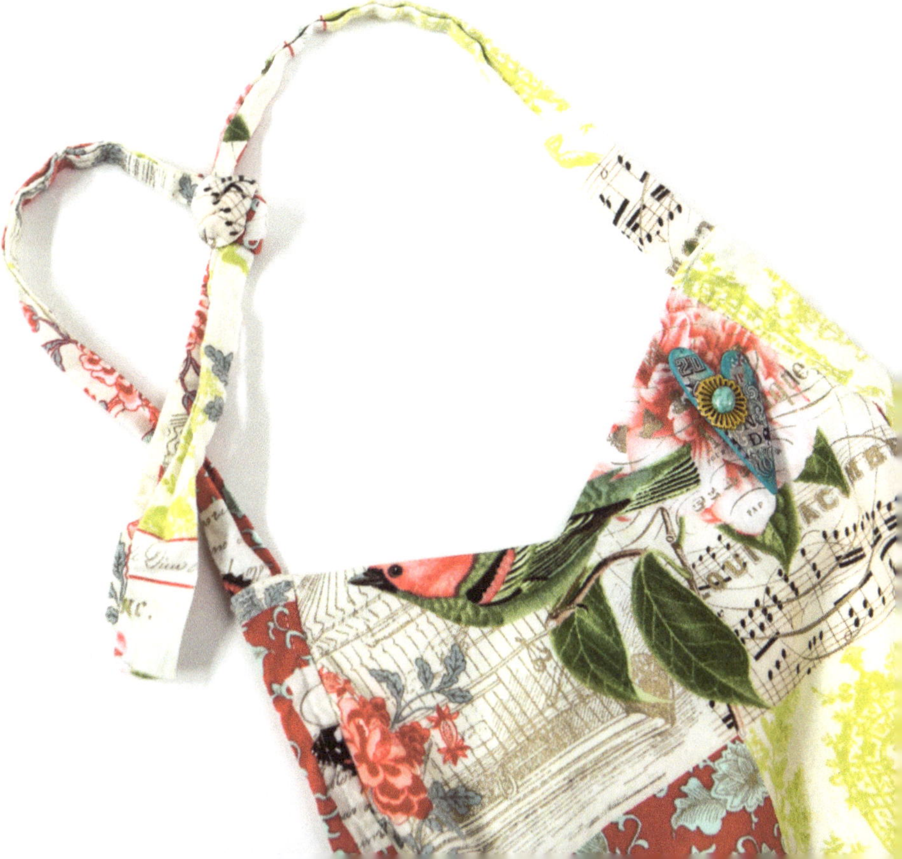

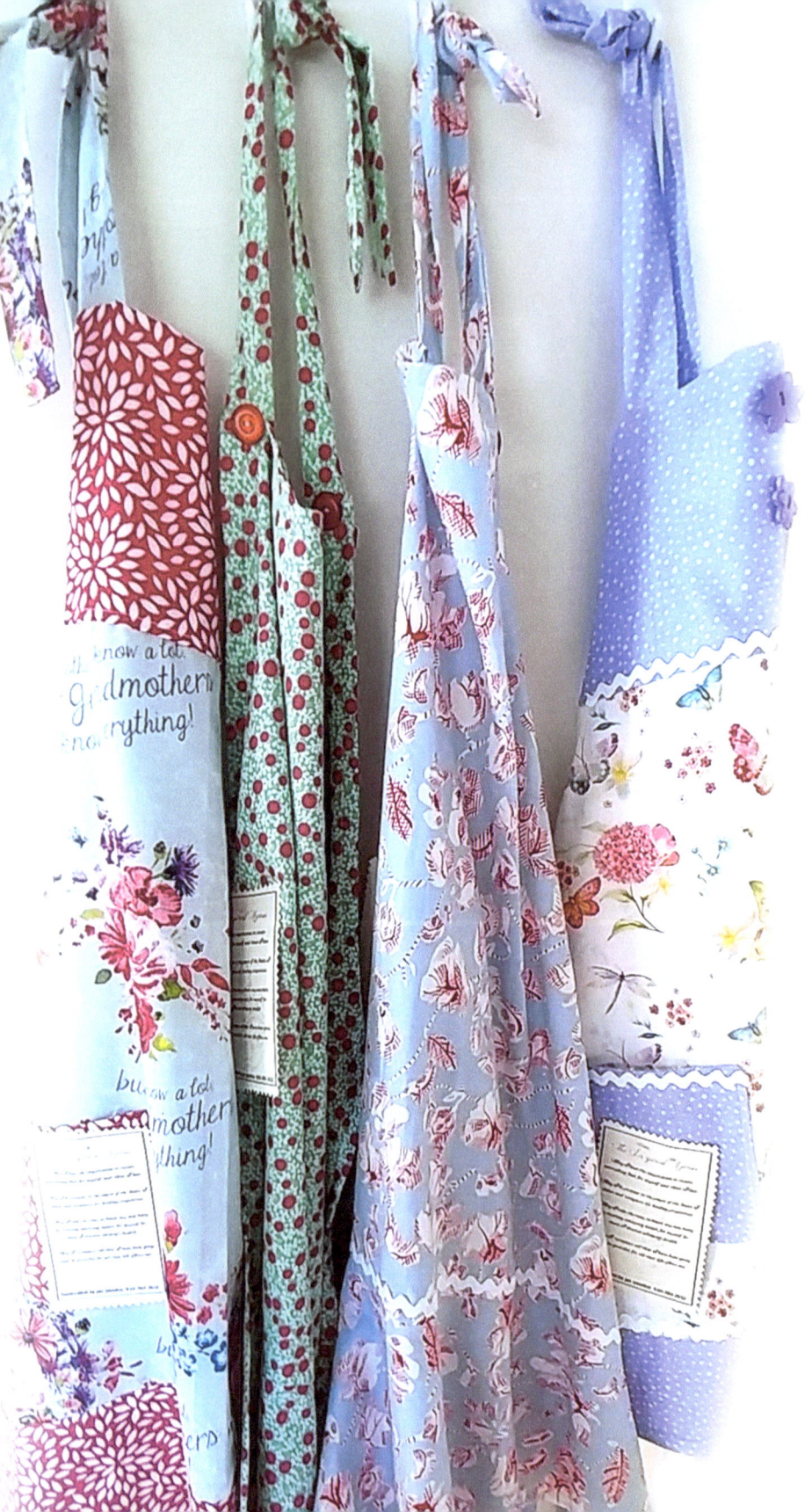

THE INSPIRED APRON
A Recipe for Life

A little book of inspiration and

recipes that feeds your mind,

body, and soul.

JAN PAVELCO
PHOTOGRAPHY BY JAN PAVELCO

Copyright © 2018 by Jan Pavelco

All rights reserved.

No part of this book may be reproduced in any form or by any electronic or mechanical means, including information storage and retrieval systems, without permission in writing from the author.

For information, contact Jan Pavelco at pavelcoj@ptd.net

The content of this book is for general informational purposes only. It is not meant to be used, nor should it be used, to diagnose or treat any medical condition or to replace the services of your physician or other healthcare provider. The advice and strategies contained in the book may not be suitable for all readers. Please consult your healthcare provider for any questions that you may have about your own medical situation. Neither the author, publisher, IIN nor any of their employees or representatives guarantees the accuracy of information in this book or its usefulness to a particular reader, nor are they responsible for any damage or negative consequences that may result from any treatment, action taken, or inaction by any person reading or following the information in this book.

To contact the author, visit

www.essenceintegratednutrition.com

ISBN-13: 978-1725167117
ISBN-10: 1725167115

Printed in the United States of America

To Logan

My most precious surprise in life. You are the reason I began

my quest for ultimate health.

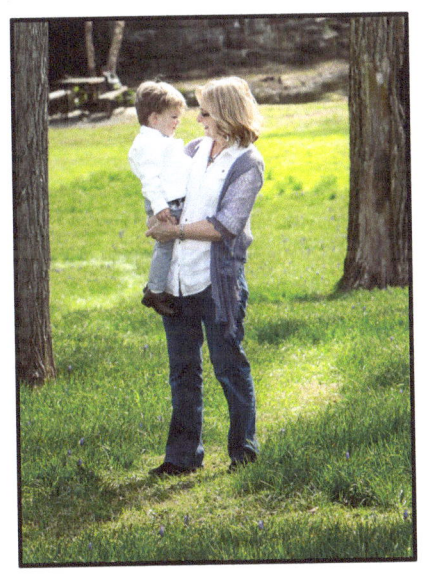

A RECIPE FOR USING THIS BOOK

Keep it handy

Turn to any page

Take a minute to read a passage

Let the spark of inspiration stir within you

Feel even better and get moving on what inspired you

Share with others

Repeat above steps as needed

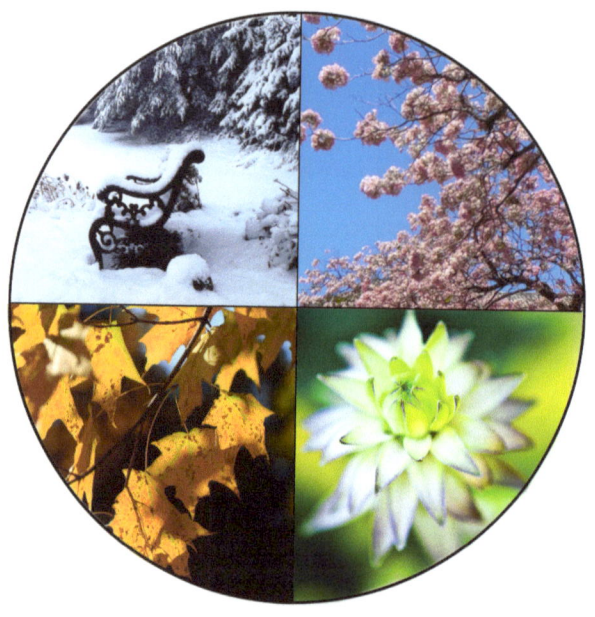

My hope is that whoever reads this little book of inspiration will have a spark ignite within them. It might be experimenting with one of the recipes in this book, or better yet, cooking fearlessly to create your own dish. My wish is that you empower yourself and those you love by the foods you choose and the way you live your life. The reflective passages are meant to be a starting point, a teaser into where your mind can wander. I want it to be a spring board for the reader. Let your mind run wild and play with all the possibilities. I want your memories to come flooding back. Each and every one of us is unique unto ourselves. No one exists like me and you, and it's up to us to make the most of every precious moment. We are never too young to start making good choices, and we are never too old to change.

Get Inspired!

Table of Contents

A Recipe for Life 1
Introduction 3
In the Light of Morning 4

SPRING 7
Take Time to Connect, Nothing to Eat, The Good Life, There's No Taste Like Home, Life Is Short

Peanut Butter Eggs 9
Free-to-be-me Yogurt 12
Cream of Mushroom and Asparagus Soup 16
Home Made Pierogies 21

SUMMER 25
Farm to Table, A Kitchen Garden, Creating Sacred Space, Home Sweet Home, Par for the Course

So Easy Vegetable Soup 30
Tomato Soup and Grilled Cheese Panini 34
Summery Zucchini Soup 38
Fresh Summer Slaw 43

AUTUMN 47
Facing the Storm, What's Eating You, Just Breathe, The Perfect Recipe

Empty the Fridge Quiche 52
Zucchini Bread 56
Mom's Apple Pie 61
How to Soak Nuts 63

WINTER 65
Ritual vs. Habit, Peeling Back the Layers, Table for One, Preserve Family Traditions, Honor a Simple Choice, At the End of the Day

White Chicken Chili 70
Sweet Potato Bisque 75
Christmas Cutout Cookies 79
Cream of Broccoli and Cheese Soup 82

IN ADDITION 87
Souper Sundays, How to Order an Apron, A Heartfelt Thank You, Favorite Gems to Shop, About the Institute for Integrative Nutrition®

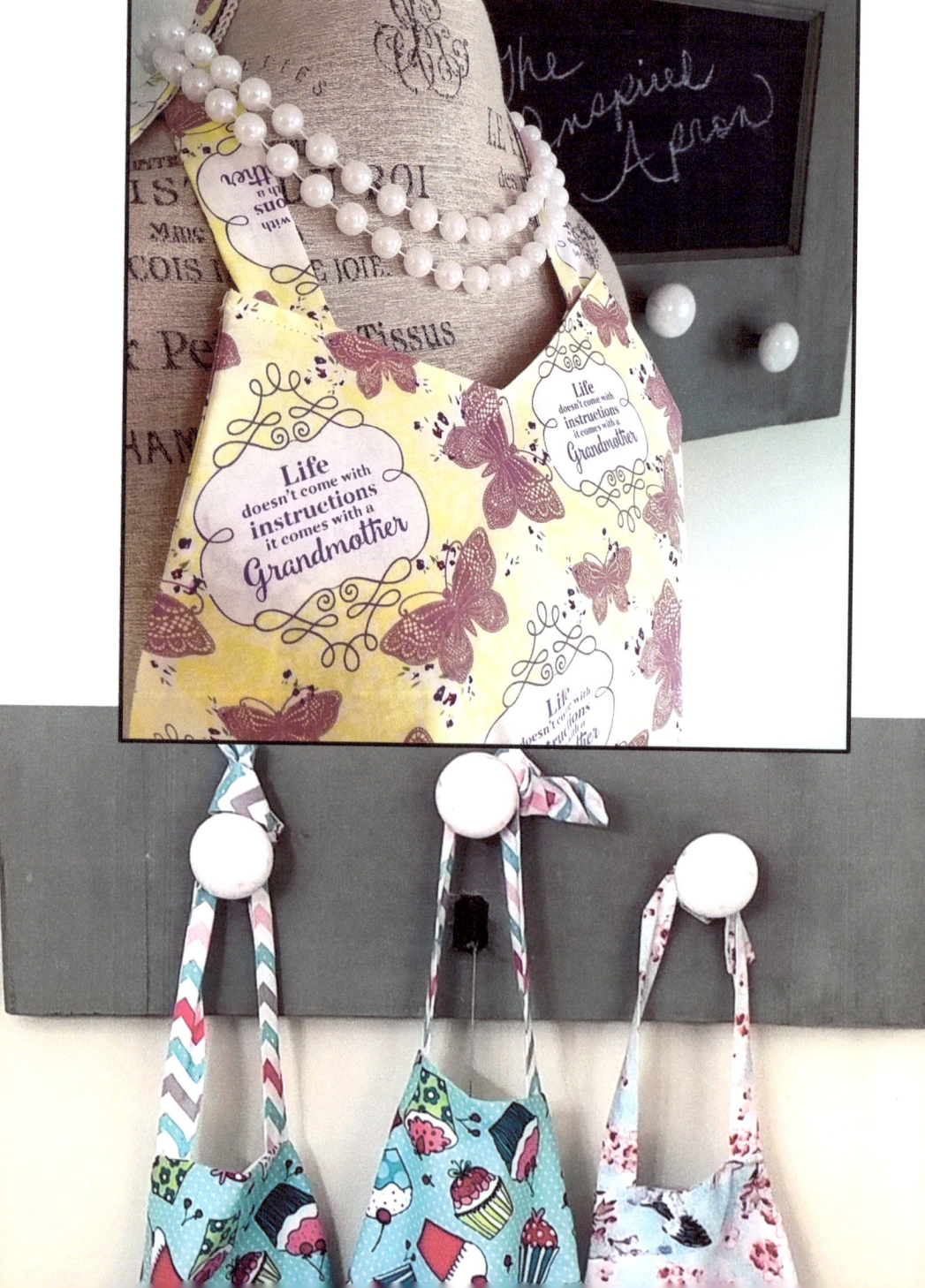

A Recipe for Life

Start where you are

Combine equal parts of faith, hope, and trust

Add a little more faith if necessary

Mix until just right

Stir in a pinch of something unexpected

Turn up the heat until it sizzles

Toss gently and make it pretty

Enjoy with friends and family

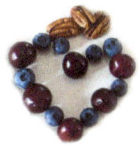

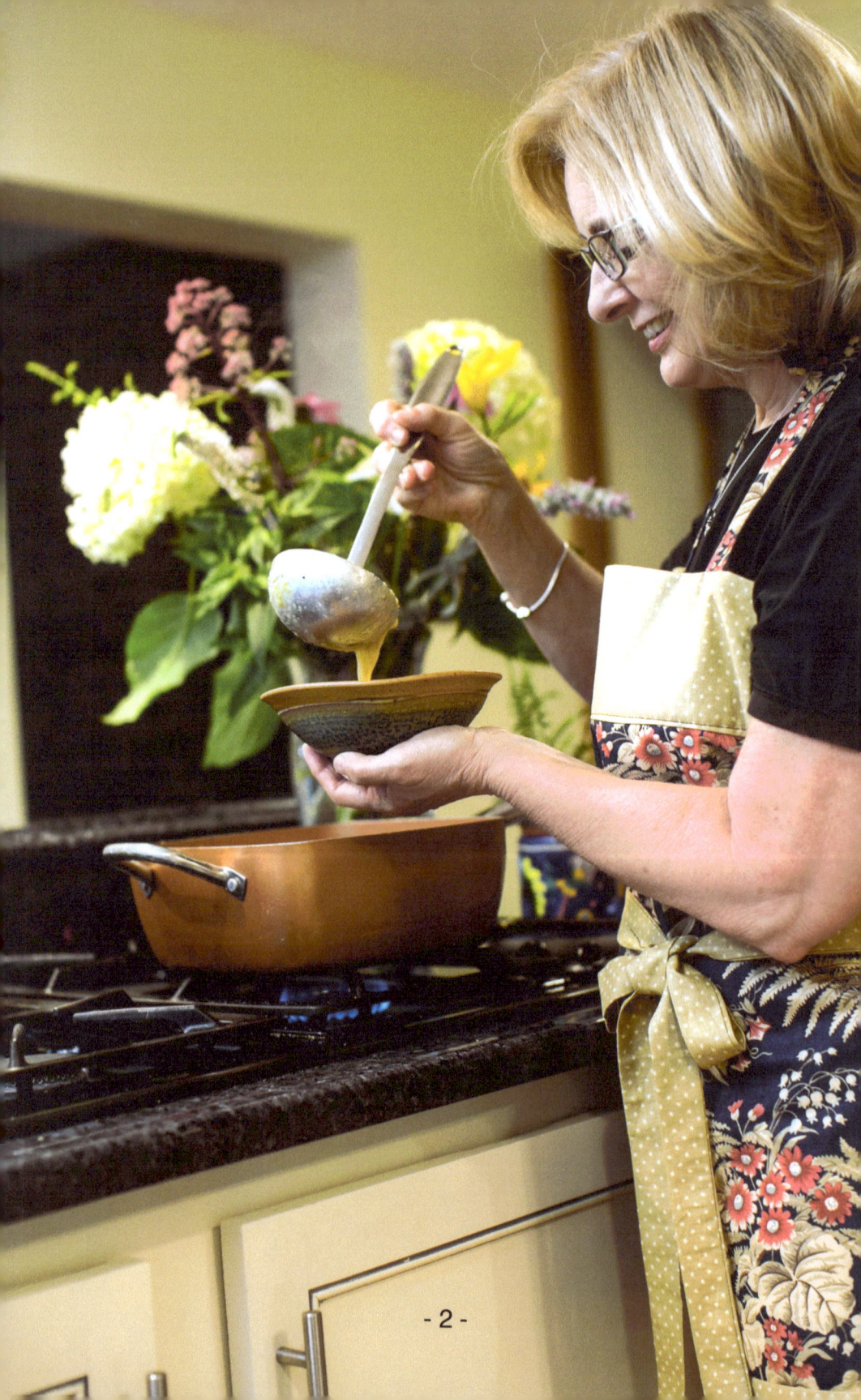

...and so it all began

It's funny how life's twists and turns takes us to places we never imagined. My connection to the power of the apron started long before I ever knew it did. Growing up, all I ever saw my mother wear was a simple house dress and an apron. A Polish mother of six children from a humble working-class family, wearing an apron was something she just did. I doubt she ever took the time to recognize its power or significance. I never gave it a second thought. Something deep inside me was recording everything though, imprinting my very DNA with something extraordinary. Little did I know, that decades later I'd be the one putting on an apron as a symbol of empowered cooking.

It started innocently enough. Make an apron. Wear it to teach a cooking class. No harm in that.... right? Then one of the classmates pointed out that, "Of course, you have to wear an apron to cook! It's what you do. You wouldn't go to a yoga class in street clothing. You'd wear yoga pants. So why would you cook without wearing an apron?" That's all it took to make the connection between how I approached the act of cooking and how the healing power of food nurtured every cell in my body.

The apron became a symbolic "touch point". Much like Buddhists use their mala beads as a connection to the spirit within, the apron became my touch point. Clark Kent had his cape, Wonder Woman had her bustier, and I had my apron.... lots of them! Each time I put one on, it signaled something within me that it was time to stop everything else and focus on the art of nourishing myself and those I loved.

I started making aprons for friends and family. Readers all over Facebook loved them and ordered them, too. I was going to inspire the world of mindful cooking one apron at a time. The ritual of draping it over my head and wrapping the strings around my waist was all it took to activate the healing power that focused, deliberate, loving preparation of food was capable of creating.

And so, the love affair with food and its power to heal began.

In the light of morning

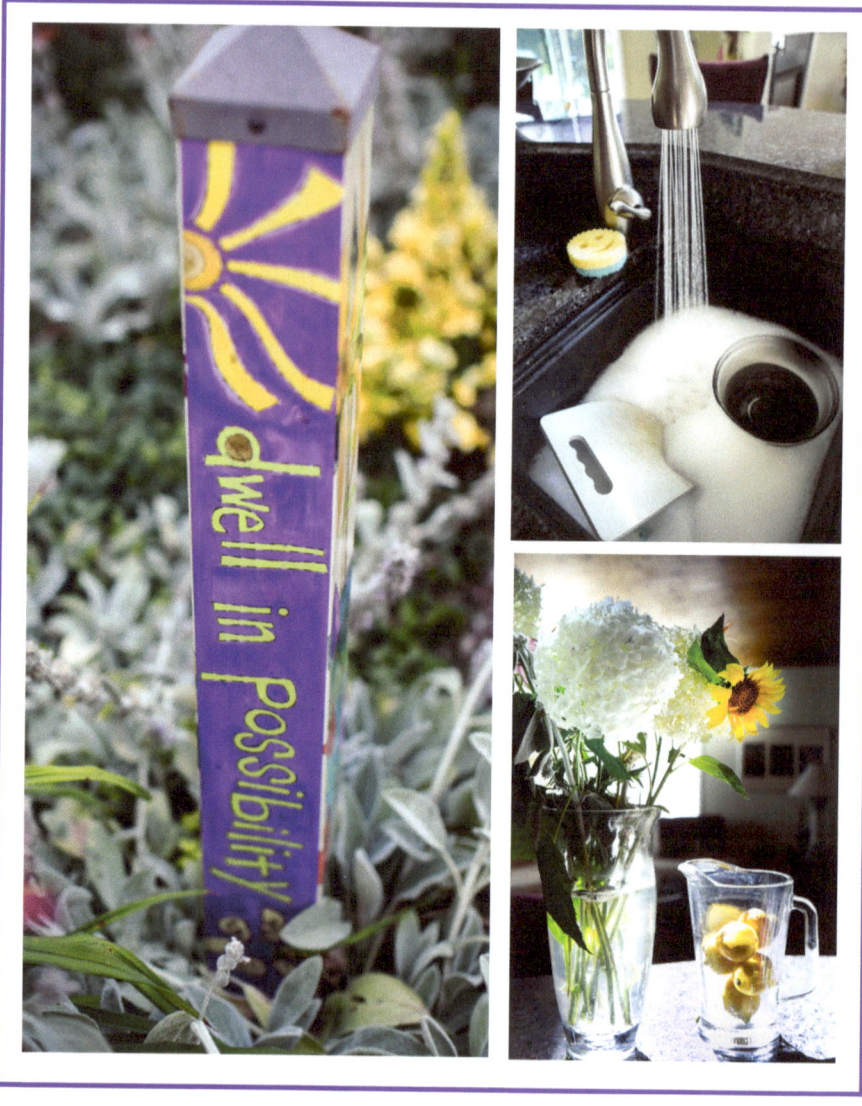

Forrest Gump once said, "Life is like a box of chocolates"; but this morning, for some strange reason, my inner voice said, "Life is like a box of Cracker Jacks". When you think you are reaching the end of the box, suddenly there's a wonderful sweet little surprise....a gift! In the past 67 years, I've had many careers: a teacher, a photographer, and now an integrative health coach. I couldn't have predicted any of these paths. I remember sitting in my community college's guidance counselor's office on orientation day. The counselor, Dave Moyer, said to me, "So you want to be a secretary?" (because that's the only thing I thought I could be without a college prep background) I said, "No, not really." "What do you want to be?" he asked. I paused. "Well, maybe I could be a teacher." My brother was a teacher. If he could do it, surely those same genes ran in me too. I'd be a business teacher because that's what I knew best from high school. "OK", he said, "A business teacher it is. Where would you like to transfer to after these two years are up?" What! Transfer! Well, where can I go? He showed me two affordable state college brochures. I picked the one that looked like it had less hills. It was settled. I was going to be a business teacher for life. And so it was for 33.73 years, and then life opened its doors to a whole new world. I often wonder what my life would be like if Dave Moyer wasn't sitting in that seat that fateful morning. That career, unbeknownst to me, laid the foundation for my present self.

None of us know what lies ahead of us or where life will take us. The twists and turns, nooks and crannies, or what we need to experience to become that little gift at the bottom of the box is never clear. No way did I ever imagine myself as a health coach and cooking instructor. The Game of Life changes everything; funny how that happens. Today there are a few things I do know for sure: breathing brings me to the present moment, caramelizing onions is like watching paint dry, there's great joy in swinging in a hammock with my grandson while telling make-believe stories about the dinosaur and the little boy, and the simple act of washing dishes should not be taken for granted. All these things become the little gems in life.

It's my hope that this book will inspire you to examine your own journey. To take time. Breathe. Play. Be grateful. Honor who you are, where you've been, and who you are becoming. We have the power to create magic in our lives, one little step at a time. Today I am many things, but most of all, today I am grateful.

Be grateful

Farm to Table

A Kitchen Garden

Creating Sacred Space

Home Sweet Home

Par for the Course

Spring

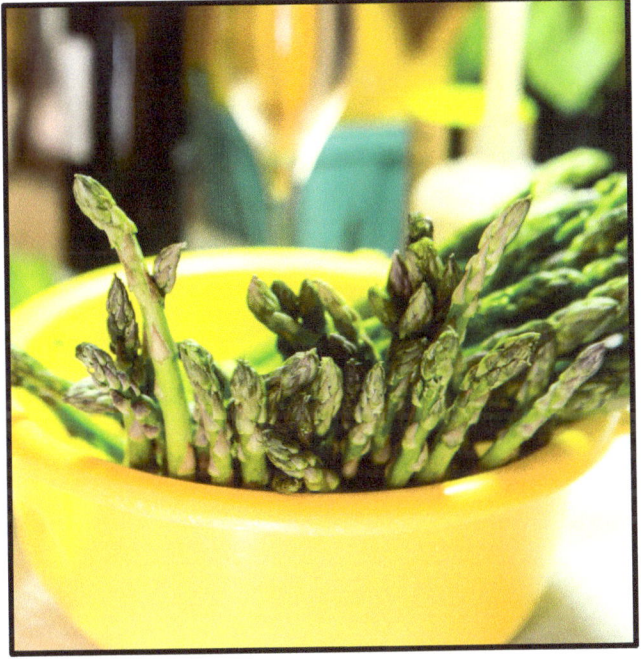

Look forward to starting something new

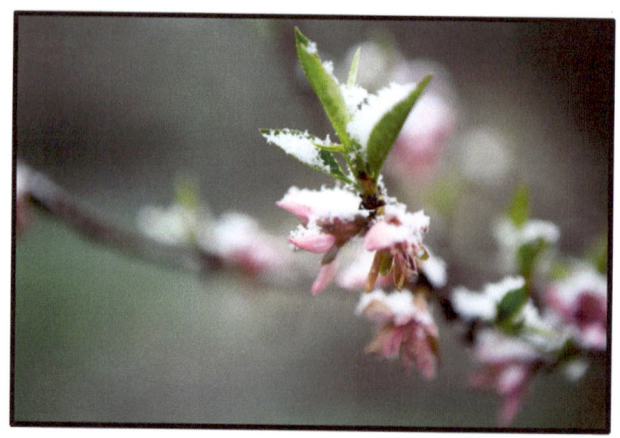

Welcome Spring

Time to wake up after a long winter's rest

Each day a little more sunshine fills our lives. Heavy winter coats get replaced with lighter jackets, and buds on trees signal that spring is just around the corner. Although we still struggle with some snow now and again, spring is a time to look forward to getting outside and being more active after a long winter's rest.

For those who celebrate Easter, this season of rebirth signals that we are waking up. Pop-up tents sell lilies and before long daffodils and tulips show up everywhere. The smell of hyacinths in the air is magical. The Easter Bunny makes an appearance, and his visit wouldn't be complete without Easter eggs. My son drops less-than-subtle hints that it's time to make peanut butter eggs. It's one of those traditions that started when he was little, and now it wouldn't seem like Easter unless I made them.

Family traditions are the cornerstone to our feeling of home, and that sense of home is such an important part of who we are today. When we think of the traditions we were part of, it brings back sweet memories of the way it was. I remember as a child going to the store to buy baby Easter chicks. Real, live baby chickens colored pink, blue, green, and purple! That would never fly now, but it was something that as a little girl I remember vividly. Look back at family traditions and enjoy them, but remember to take time to make new ones too.

Peanut Butter Eggs

There are no words for how delicious these peanut butter eggs are. I'm not making any claim about them being totally healthy, but I do know that they are sooooo much better than any store-bought version. I get to eat one or two to celebrate Easter and then gift them away to friends and family who love them.

You're gonna need:

1 cup softened butter

10 oz. cream cheese

2 tsp. vanilla

24 oz. peanut butter

32 oz. powdered sugar

Here's what to do:

Beat all the above ingredients together until smooth and creamy. Using your hands, scoop up small amounts of the creamy mixture and roll them into small egg shaped balls. Place the rolled eggs on parchment paper and put them in the freezer to get really cold. Make sure they don't touch each other and are only one layer thick.

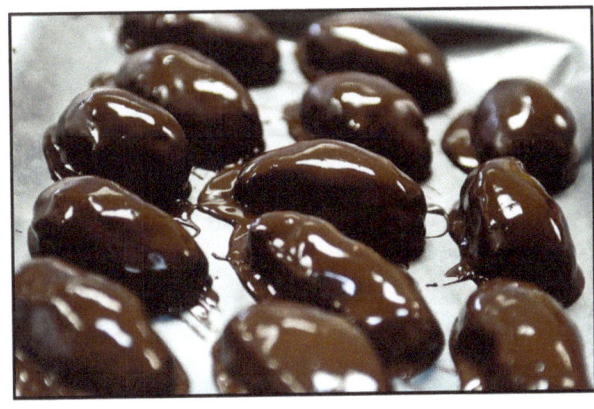

Melt two boxes of baker's chocolate squares in a double boiler. I add a little chunk (about 1") of paraffin wax to help make it glossier. You can control the amount of sugar in the coating by selecting either milk chocolate, semi-sweet or bitter. The higher the percentage of cocoa, the less sugar content.

Using a long skewer to hold the eggs, dip the frozen egg in the melted chocolate and then immediately place it on a parchment lined cookie sheet. Place the sheet back in the freezer until the chocolate hardens. These treats can be frozen for a long time and taken out as a heavenly bite right from the freezer.

Take Time to Connect
Trusting the Divine within

A statue of a frog sits at the edge of my tiny pond. Day in, day out, season after season, never moving a muscle. Deep in meditation and prayer, this frog doesn't let anything disturb him. It rains on him, snow covers him, and heat bakes him. He still sits as still as can be with single-minded focus. It's so easy for him, duh..... he's a statue. It's his job. Someone created him to be a reminder to us humans that just once in a while we need to do the same.

Spirituality is one of the four key factors that play a vital role in our overall health. It's important to understand that the primary sources of health are the balance of career, physical activity, relationships, and spirituality. Food is actually secondary to these four. This is the keystone of the teachings of the Institute for Integrative Nutrition® where I studied. But long before I was a student at IIN, I knew the importance of a spiritual connection to the Divine.

Whether you call it God, Buddha, Allah, or Yahweh, teachings tell us that "all is one". Our connection to spirit, in my own humble opinion, is much different than the religion we were born into. Whether we belong to a church or not and how often we attend, if we do belong, is irrelevant. I know a lot of people who go to church every Sunday only out of obligation, and then I also know so many people who never enter a church yet are extremely connected to their faith. Isn't it interesting how the term faith is used to describe a religion. Google describes faith as "complete trust or confidence in someone or something". Once again, this complete trust in the Divine can be experienced anywhere. No church wall can confine it. It goes as deep as our soul allows it to. This "faith" is tested continuously, and it's our ability to stay the course that gives us our greatest strength.

Like the frog at the edge of the pond, it's our job to tap into our faith and stay centered and calm when life challenges us and to give thanks when life is good.

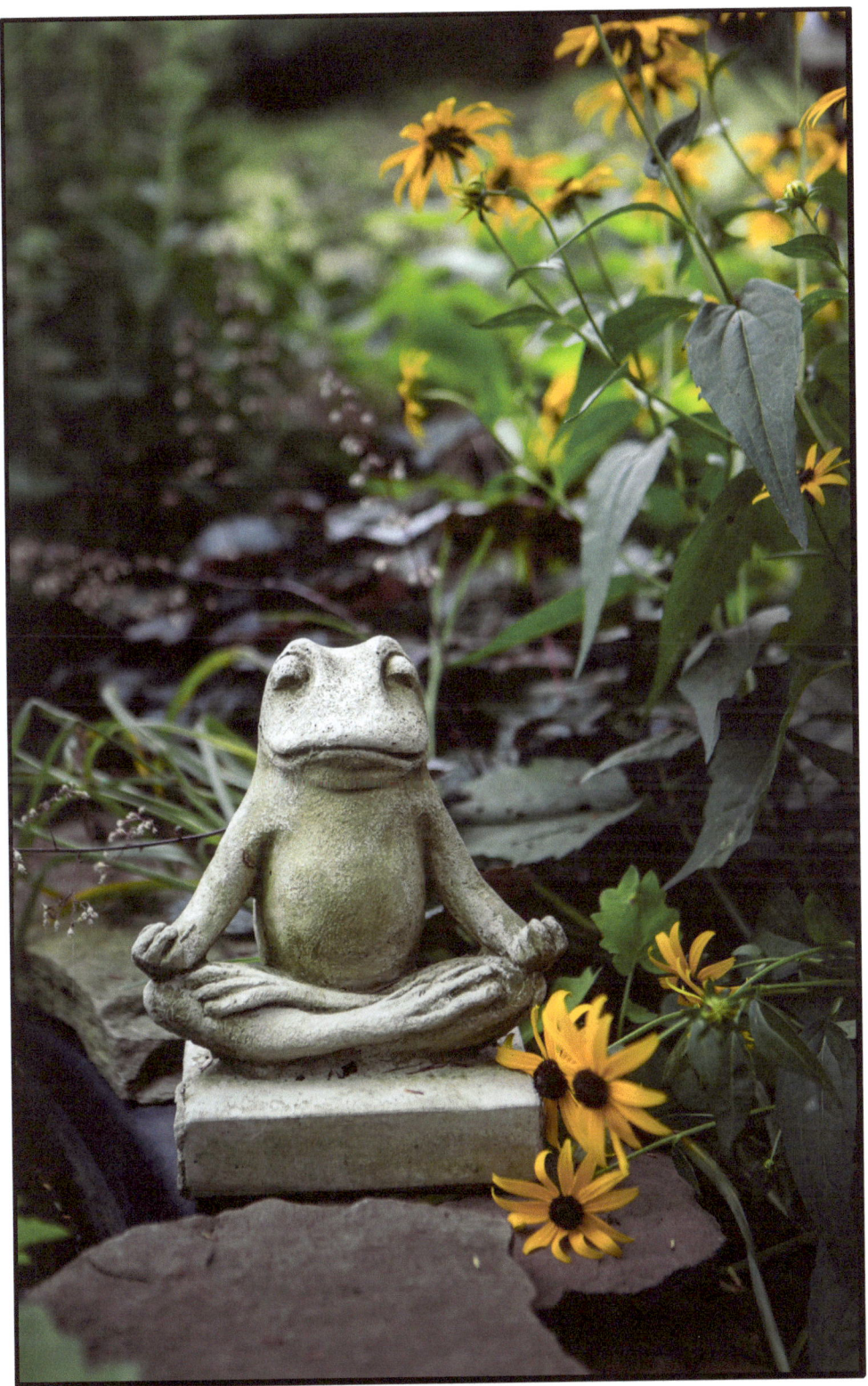

Free-to-be-me Yogurt

The world of breakfast food can easily be full of landmines of unhealthy carbs and sugars. Cereal, bagels, and donuts, yikes! That's what so many people grab on their way out the door. By taking matters into your own hands, you have the freedom and power to create a healthy and nourishing start to your day. One of my favorite go-to options is to create my own bowl of goodness.

The first step is to choose a yogurt that isn't full of sugar. Easier said than done. I'm in love with the brand So Delicious dairy free coconut milk yogurt alternative. It has less than one gram of sugar and is the perfect base to build on. After that, it's so easy to layer on tons of goodness. Add fresh berries that are in season, your favorite nuts or a dollop of almond butter, and a sprinkling of chia seeds and hemp hearts.

The bowl is your playground, so go for it. Don't hold back on what you can add. You have permission to explore, play, create and most of all enjoy eating!

Food for Thought!

Chia seeds are rich in antioxidants, which help fight free radical damage in the body. It's a great source of plant protein. These tiny seeds are about 14 percent protein; and not only that, chia seeds have more calcium than most dairy products. Just one tablespoon will provide you with 100 percent of your daily requirement for omega-3 ALA. Studies also show that chia seeds can significantly lower blood pressure. The possibilities of where to incorporate chia seeds are endless. Sprinkling them on yogurt and salads is a perfect way to use them.

If you are a smoothie drinker, chia seeds are an excellent addition to your mix.

> "
> One man's food is another man's poison as they say, so listen to your body. If you are allergic to nuts, then it's a no-brainer to keep them off your list of ingredients! The same goes for fruit. If you have sugar issues, be sure to choose wisely.
> "

Hemp hearts add a delicious nutty flavor and are full of omegas 3 and 6, magnesium, iron, and manganese (just to mention a few). Hemp hearts are a powerhouse of protein with next to no sugar. It's best to choose nonGMO organic whenever possible.

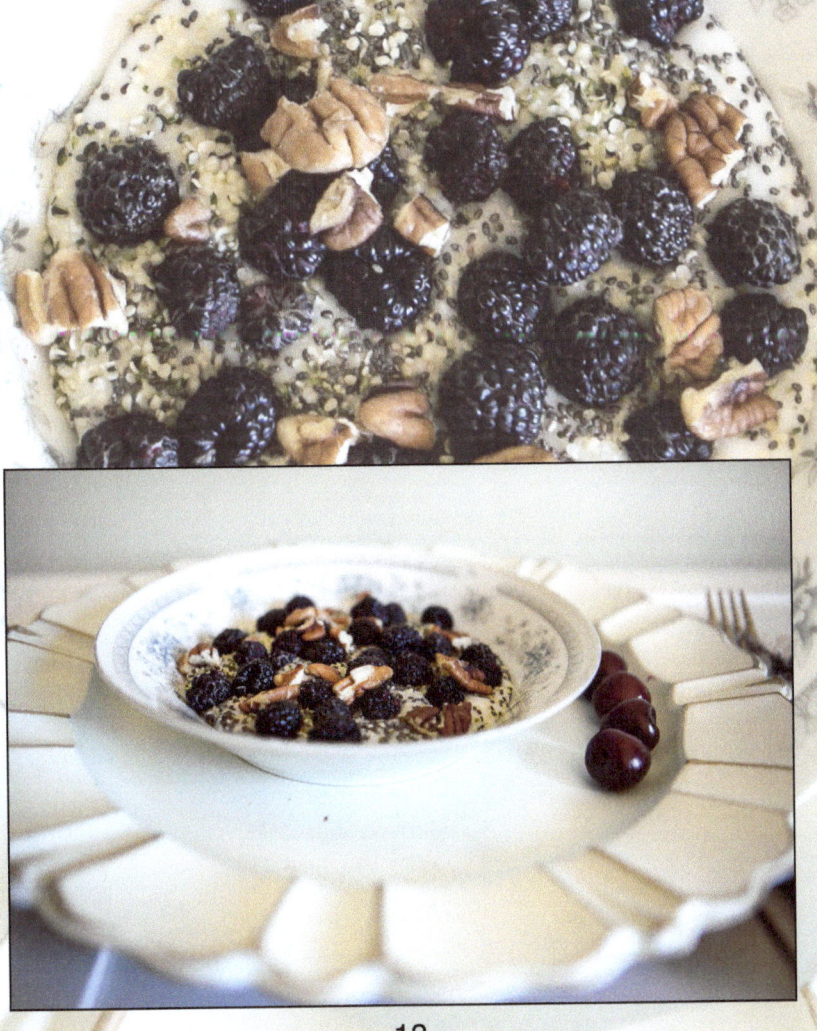

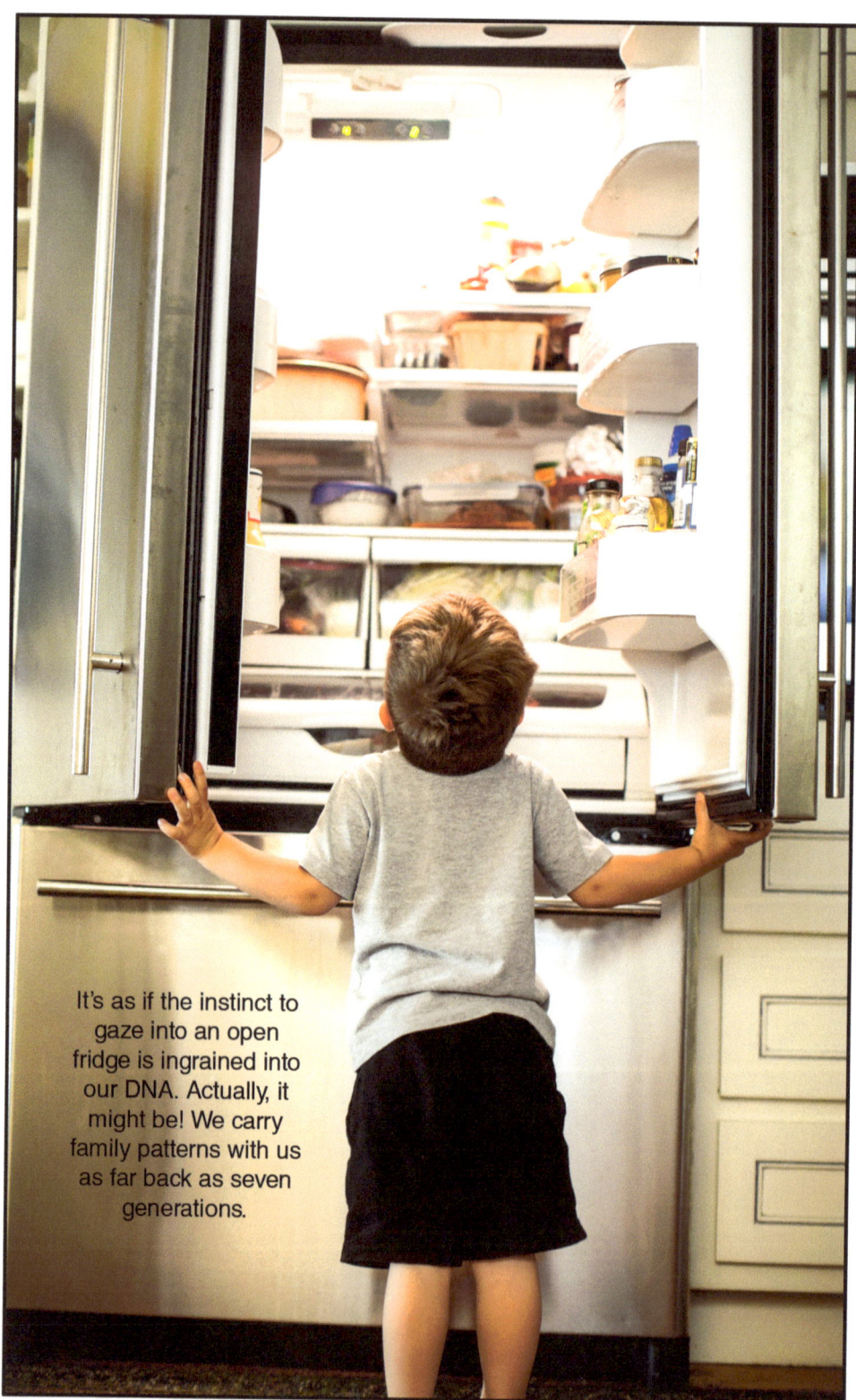

It's as if the instinct to gaze into an open fridge is ingrained into our DNA. Actually, it might be! We carry family patterns with us as far back as seven generations.

Nothing to eat....
Think again! Easy go-to healthy foods

Is there anyone alive who hasn't opened the refrigerator or pantry and stared with glazed-over eyes at "absolutely nothing to eat"? Of course there's something to eat! But is it what you want, is there time to make it, and is it healthy? These are the loaded questions that can derail even the best of intentions when it comes to sticking to a healthy eating plan. We stare into the fridge looking for answers.

One solution is to have healthy options on hand that will stay fresh for a long time. Stock food that is loaded with healthy fats and nutrients. Nuts, olives, avocado, cheese, and eggs are foods that will satisfy you. Add a piece of fruit like an apple and you are ready to go.

NUTS: contain heart-healthy unsaturated fats. They contain protein, fiber, and plant stanols, which may help lower cholesterol, and antioxidants including vitamin E.

OLIVES: are very high in vitamin E and other powerful antioxidants. Studies show that they are good for the heart, and may protect against osteoporosis and cancer.

AVOCADOS: are a great source of vitamins C, E, K, and B-6, as well as riboflavin, niacin, folate, magnesium, and potassium. They also provide lutein, beta-carotene, and omega-3 fatty acids.

HARD BOILED EGGS: are a good source of high quality protein. The whites are rich sources of selenium, vitamin D, B6, B12 and minerals such as zinc, iron, and copper. I love red beet eggs!

CHEESE: contains calcium, protein, phosphorus, zinc, vitamin A and vitamin B12. Easy does it, though, moderation is key.

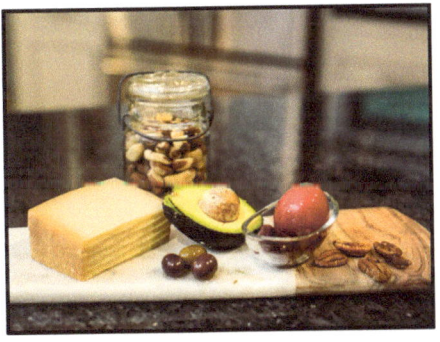

EASY GRAB-N-EAT FOODS

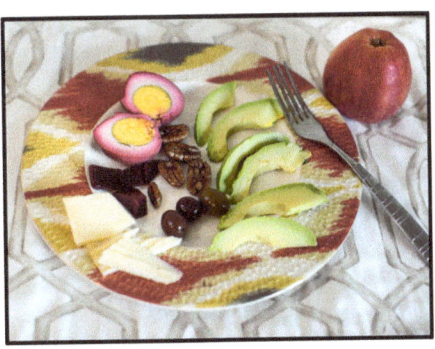

Breakfast, lunch, or even dinner.... this plate is both nourishing and satisfying. Add greens, and presto: You have a salad.

Cream of Mushroom
and Asparagus Soup

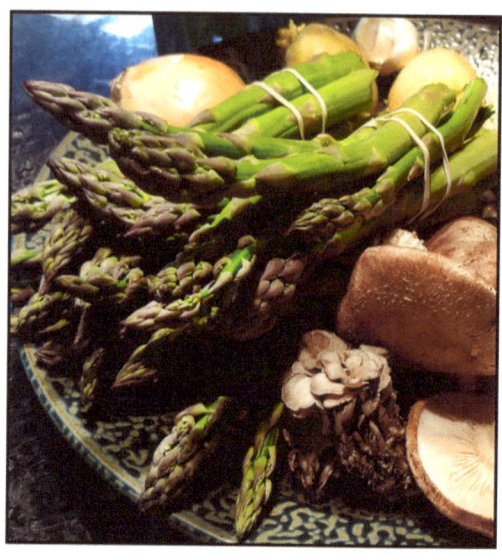

You're gonna need:

3 slices of bacon
1/4 cup butter
3 stalks celery, chopped
1 onion, diced
3 tablespoons flour
6 cups chicken broth
1 potato, peeled and diced
1 pound fresh asparagus, tips set aside and stalks chopped
salt and pepper to taste
2 cups fresh mushrooms, diced
3/4 cup half-and-half cream

Here's what to do:

1. Place bacon in a frying pan and cook until it is evenly brown and looks crispy. When bacon is done, place it on a paper towel to absorb excess grease. Keep 1 tablespoon of the bacon grease to use in the recipe. Discard remaining bacon grease from fry pan, but don't wash the pan! We will use it later in the recipe. Crumble bacon when cool and set aside.

2. Melt butter and the 1 tablespoon of bacon drippings in a deep pot over medium heat. Add the celery and onion and sauté until onion is translucent, about 4 minutes.

3. Add flour into the mixture, stir and cook for about 1 minute. Then add the chicken broth and bring it to a boil. Add potato and chopped asparagus stalks, reserving the asparagus tips for later. Season with salt and ground black pepper.

4. Lower the heat and simmer for about 20 minutes or until potatoes are fully cooked. Using an immersion blender, puree the soup until it is smooth and creamy.

5. Use the fry pan that the bacon was cooked in to sauté the mushrooms and asparagus tips. Add a little butter if necessary to keep mushrooms and asparagus from sticking. Sauté until mushrooms are nice and brown.

6. Stir mushrooms, asparagus tips, and half-and-half cream into the pureed soup. Cook until thoroughly heated and get ready to say "Yum".

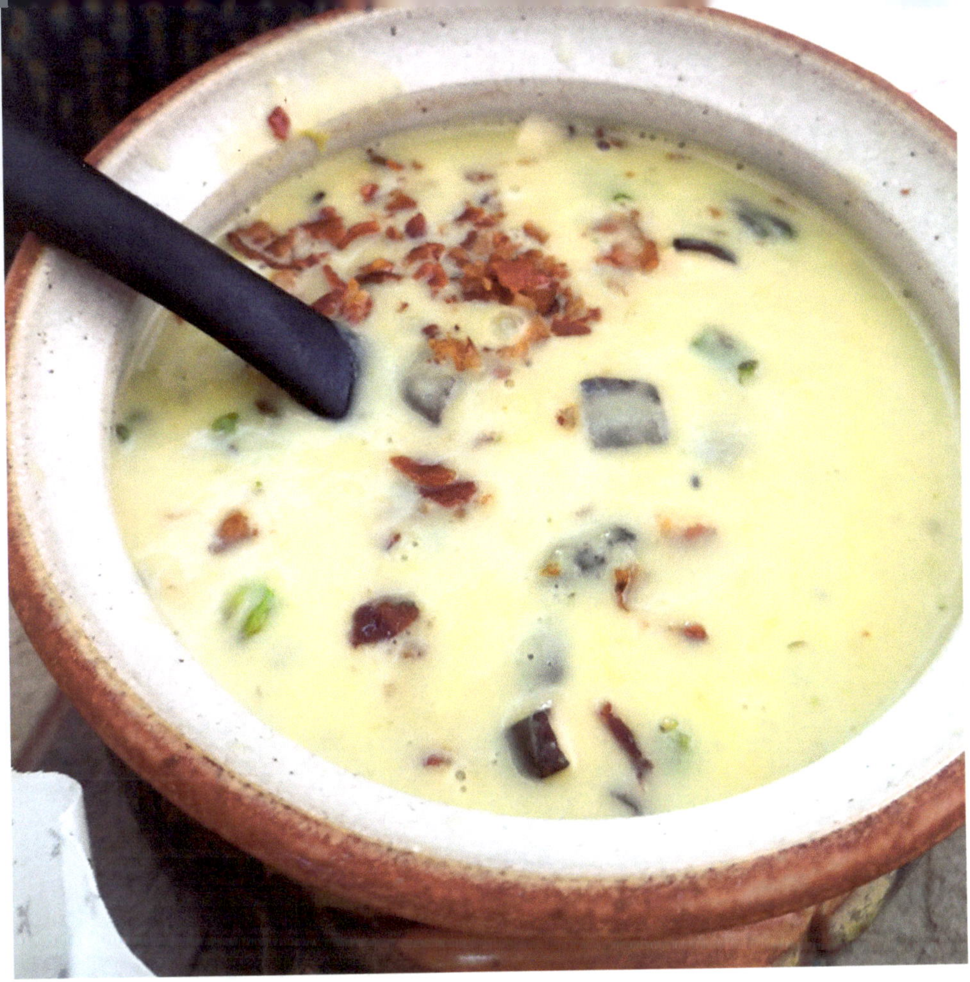

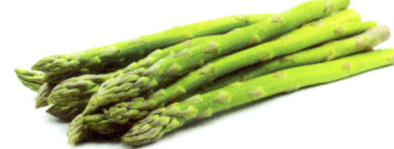

Asparagus is high in vitamin K, which is the blood clotting vitamin. Vitamin K can also improve our bone health. Studies have demonstrated that vitamin K can not only increase bone mineral density in osteoporotic people, but it can actually reduce fracture rates. Asparagus also contains the nutrient inulin, which does not break down in our digestive tract. Instead, it passes undigested to our large intestines, where it becomes a food source for good, healthy bacteria. Good bacteria are responsible for better nutrient absorption, a lower risk of allergies, and a lower risk of colon cancer.

Food for Thought!

The Good Life
It's just a state of mind

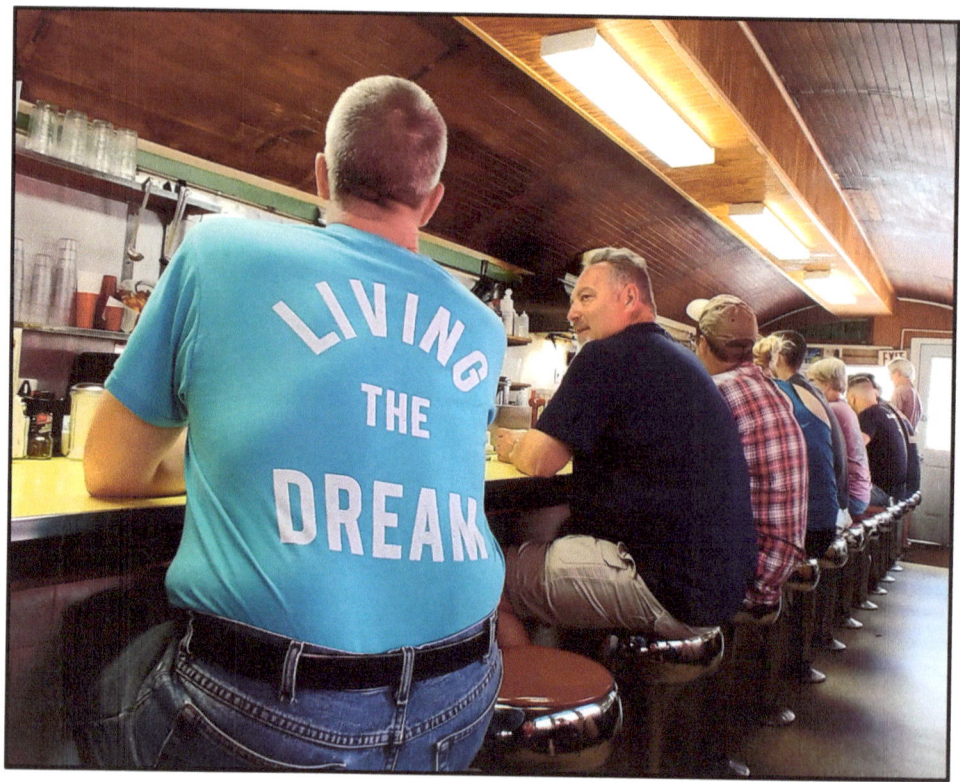

We've heard all the sayings a thousand times: Make every moment count, Live for today, Here today gone tomorrow, Count your blessings, Live the good life. Well, what exactly is the "good life"? For most of us, it's not living the lifestyle of the rich and famous. Can't you just hear the voice of that TV announcer in your head when you hear that phrase.

One Friday morning my friend and I were having the most outrageous omelet at a little diner in Kutztown called Letterman's. To the locals of this town and surrounding area, Letterman's is famous for its down-home atmosphere and meal portions that can feed a small village. It's the kind of place where, if you go there often enough, everyone knows your name. Nostalgic and homey, it's the place where you can chat with friends, family or the guy on the stool next to you. For a moment, you forget about what's happening in the world. You can eat the most gigantic breakfast that fills you up for almost the entire day. But is it the size of the breakfast alone that fills you up for the day, or is that just part of it? Feeding the body actual food is such a small part of feeling fully nourished. It's really only secondary to what our mind, body, and soul need to be completely healthy. What's primary are things like our relationships, our fulfillment in our career, our spiritual connection, and how we move our body throughout the day. It makes total sense if you think about it.

Once we make the connection that everything is interconnected and dependent on each other, then all of a sudden living the good life takes on a whole new meaning when you strive for that balance in life. It's not only noticing the little things and being grateful for them, it's doing the little things as well. Something as simple as holding the door open for someone as you walk into that diner can make life a little easier for someone, if just for the moment. It's the second cup of coffee sipped at a leisurely pace, it's being able to open your wallet and finding enough money in there to add an extra dollar to the tip. Yes, and sometimes "Living the Dream" is just saying yes to an omelet built for two.

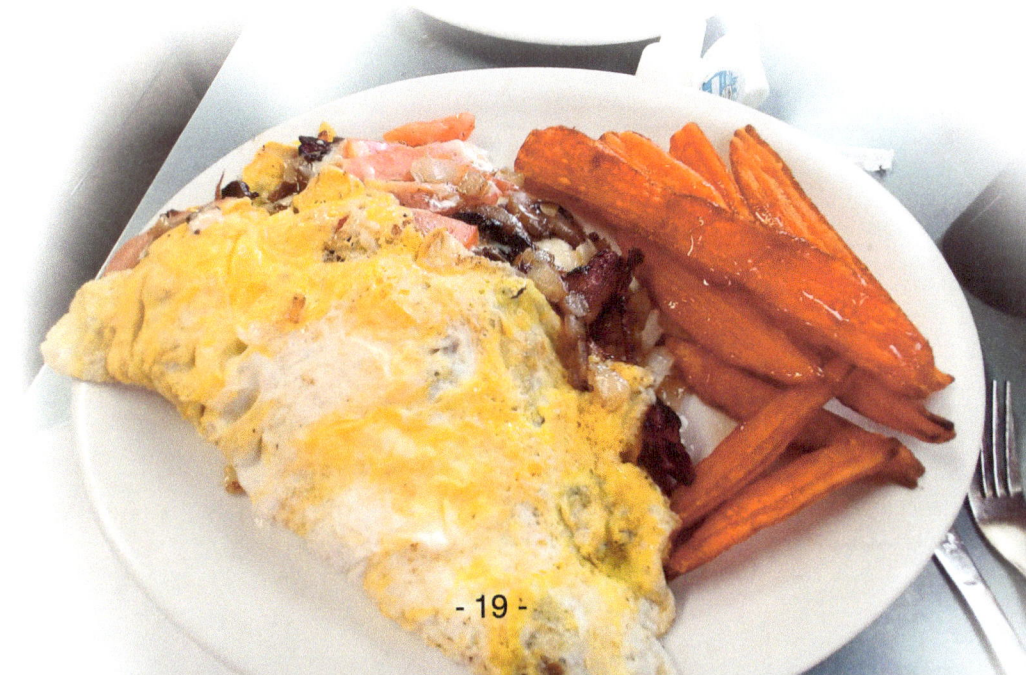

There's No Taste Like Home

Family recipes pay respect to our heritage

How many of us have had the experience of "going home" as a grown adult and opening the fridge, looking in the cookie jar, or sniffing for something good that was just cooked? Even though those days are long gone, there are still those emotional ties that have me seeking the comfort of food from my childhood.

As adults, and now in charge of our own health and wellbeing, it's those deep-rooted subconscious connections that often drive what we eat, how we cook, and what we crave, especially when we are stressed. Some of us are mothers and grandmothers now, and we are the ones who set the memories for our children. My own son reminds me at the start of each season when it's time for apple pie, Christmas cookies, homemade peanut butter eggs at Easter, and the list goes on. When we take time to honor our roots and connect with family traditions, something magical happens. We activate our DNA's memories, and that often takes us back to a time we thought we forgot. We breathe deeper, soaking in the smells and sounds from our childhood. I remember my mother and I making pierogies together. The gentle kneading of dough and the feel of the rolling pin in my hands, come flooding back now that I make them on my own.

So, why is it so important to take time to reconnect and honor our past? First of all, it feeds our soul and that alone can put us on the path to health. Life is crazier now. We grab the easiest meal possible as we dash out the door on the way to some meeting or practice. We barely take time to chew! It's no wonder that the health of today's family suffers. So, what's the best way to truly honor our family roots? The answer can be as easy as simply reconnecting to them with a family recipe. It's one meal at a time, taking time to slow down, chop, smell, and taste. It's our turn to create the memories that will be passed down to the next generation. In honoring our past, we honor our future. One healthy meal at a time.

Homemade Pierogi

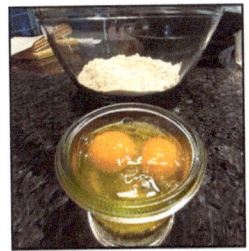

POTATO FILLING:
    Make mashed potatoes in your usual way and add at least one cup of grated cheese. It can be all one type, like American, or a combination of several cheeses. It's all according to your own preference. The potato filling should be cooled before making the pierogi.

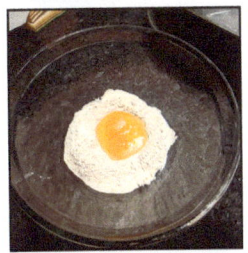

DOUGH INGREDIENTS:
2 cups flour; 1/4 tsp. salt
2 eggs
approx. 1/8 c. water

    Using a large mixing bowl, combine flour and salt. Put eggs with water in the center of the flour. Begin to knead it with your hands to form a dough. Add more flour if it still sticks to your fingers. This dough can be rolled right away. Roll out in flour. Cut into squares and fill with potato filling.

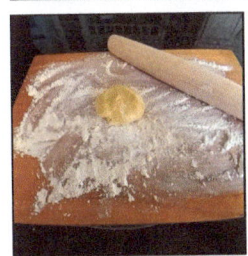

    Pinch edges tight when folding dough together. If the edges don't seal, dip your fingers in water and wet the edges to help it seal. Drop a few of the pierogi in boiling water. When they float to the top, they are done. (about 2 minutes). Sauté in butter to finish them off.

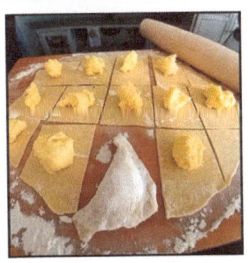

    Pierogies can be frozen. Just make sure you use some melted butter to coat them before they go into freezer bags. This will help to keep them from sticking together. To make frozen pierogies, just drop them in boiling water for about 4 minutes, drain, and then sauté them until lightly golden. They are delicious with fried onions and sour cream.

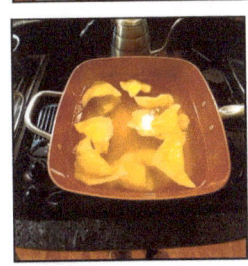

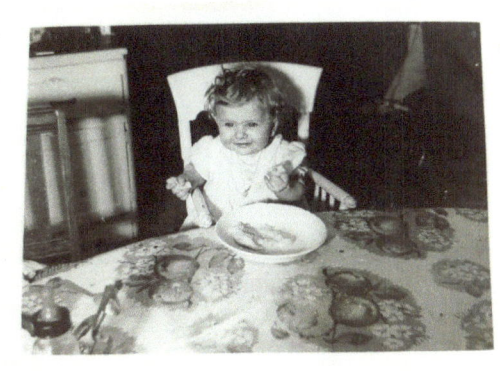
Even at 7 months old, I loved pierogies

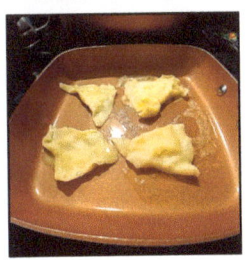

Life Is Short

Be present to every moment

A butterfly flutters from flower to flower, enjoying the sweet nectar of each flower. Moving here and there, landing for just a moment, long enough to savor the sweet taste; it takes a breath, and then it's off again. Elusive. I'm sure it probably never looks back on when it was a caterpillar, during those days of just creeping along inch by inch, waiting for the day it could just fly. And I'm not sure if it's thinking about how short its life is now that it can fly. Bold and beautiful, expansive wings that float on air, this little guy is enjoying every moment.

Now that I'm older, I think more about how much time is left. How many "good" years before the body is shot to hell, as they say. My older sister always says to me, "Enjoy it now. Getting old is no fun." I'm sure there's some truth in that; but if we worry about the future too much, there's no way that we can be fully present to enjoy the gifts of the present.

Many years ago, I traveled to Peru where I studied with two wise Shamans. Our group would sit in a circle on top of some mountain top and listen to their words of wisdom. Over and over again they would say, "Just ask yourself: who I am?" And then if that wasn't enough of a task, they'd say, "And then ask yourself, who is asking 'who I am'? I can still hear their voices in my head, in that endearing Peruvian accent. Rubin would say, "Enjoy the moment. It is a gift; that's why they call it the present."

We know that the only constant in life is change. How we adapt to those changes is a mission all unto itself. Buddhists would call it letting go of attachment. They teach that most of our suffering is caused when we put too much expectation on something. We are more attached to the outcome instead of enjoying the process. I'm not sure what that butterfly expects, or if it thinks about tomorrow at all. But what I do know for sure is that in the moment my camera's shutter captured its journey, it was simply beautiful.

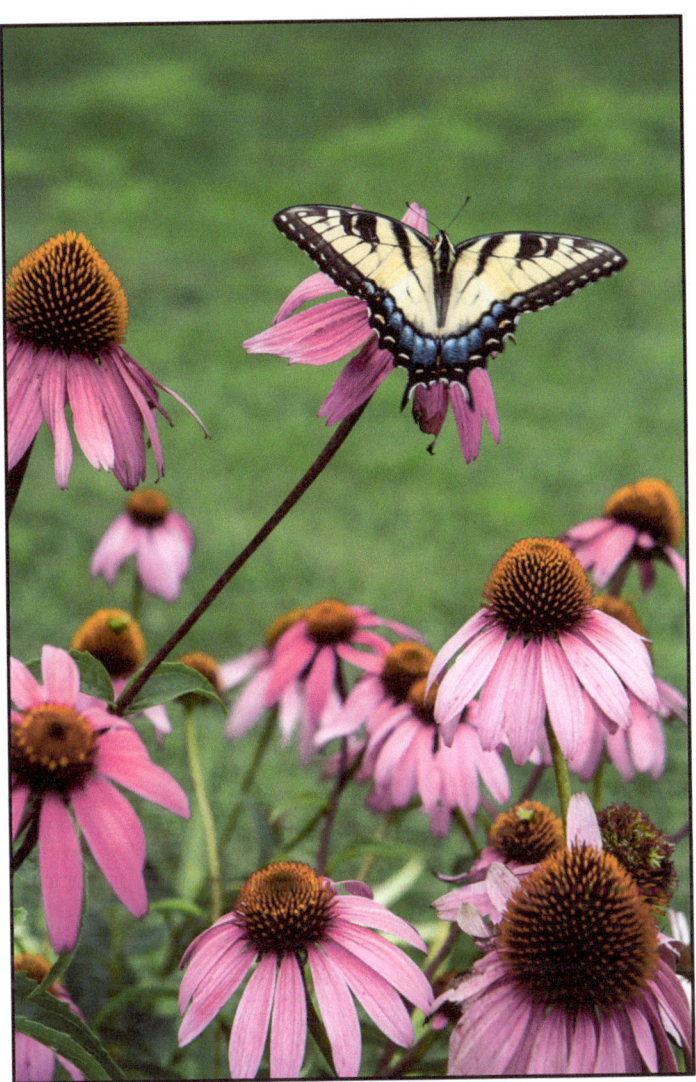

May all sentient beings have
happiness and the causes of happiness;

May all sentient beings be free from
suffering and the causes of suffering;

May all sentient beings never be separated from
the happiness that knows no suffering;

May all sentient beings abide in equanimity,
free from attachment and anger that holds
some close and others distant.

The Four Immeasurables - Tibetan Buddhism

Farm to Table

A Kitchen Garden

Creating Sacred Space

Home Sweet Home

Par for the Course

Summer

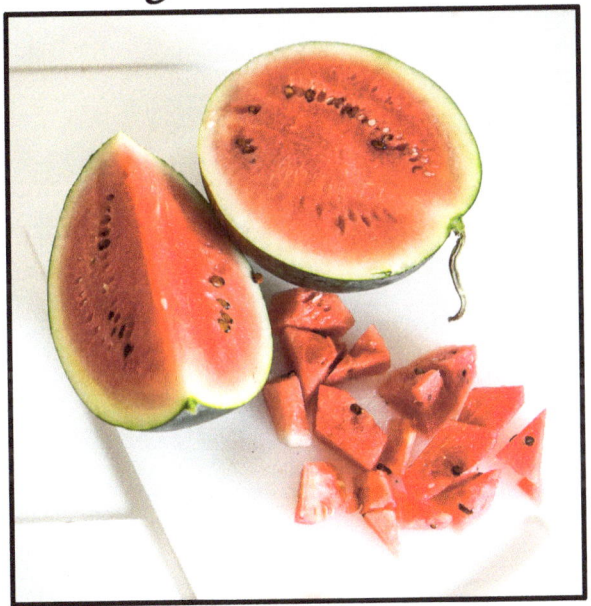

Dive into something really juicy

Awww..... Sweet Summer

Summertime, and the livin' is easy. It's the time of year we all wait for. Long days, warm nights, flip flops and fresh fruit. In the Northeast, the seasons are so different from each other; and that difference means that we need to really pay attention to what our body needs in each season. As opposed to winter, when our body craves warm comfort foods, summer signals our bodies to crave foods that naturally cool us off. Think about it. Watermelon, cool and hydrating, always tastes best in summer. We get to experience what "real" tomatoes actually taste like. We crave things like BLT sandwiches, tomato and cucumber salad, or a sweet cherry tomato right off the vine. Oh, and what about corn on the cob? How sweet is that! Unfortunately, with all the GMO corn being grown, the challenge to find organic non-GMO is tricky. Thank goodness for people like The Good Farm where organic corn is one of their crops.

It doesn't take a rocket scientist to understand our craving for ice cream, either. For me, this is one of those urges that I really have to temper. I'd eat it every day in the summer if I could. As delicious as many summery foods are, making choices that

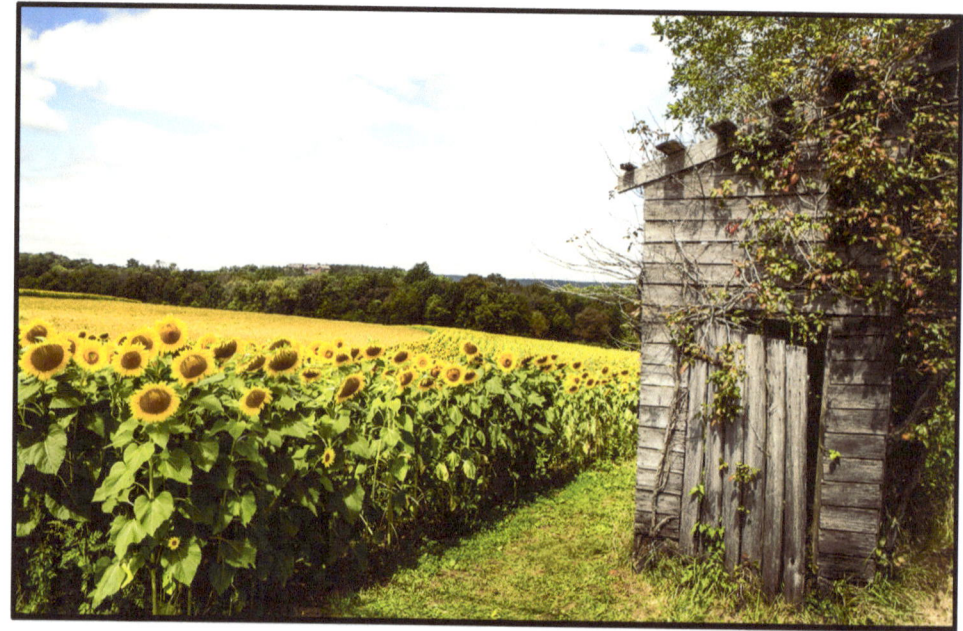

honor what our body can handle can be challenging. If someone has a blood sugar issue, then things like ice cream and all those delicious but sugary fruits are not the best choices. Those suffering from arthritis or any inflammatory condition would be better off without all those nightshade vegetables. Goodbye eggplant, peppers and tomatoes. Is nothing sacred? If you are so lucky to have both blood sugar and inflammation problems.... well let's not even go there! That's the boat I'm in, unfortunately. It is challenging, but I try to stick to the 90/10 rule. Eat what is best for the body 90 percent of the time, and then the other 10 percent of the time can be just a little indulgent for special occasions.

Summer's also a time to be more active. Physical activity is one of the primary factors in maintaining a healthy body. Once again, you can eat all the right foods, but if you are living life by watching TV or scrolling through other people's lives on Facebook, you're not going to be totally healthy. People are out everywhere doing what they've been waiting all year to do. Fishing, biking, swimming, hiking, golfing, gardening, kayaking; the choices are endless. Make the choice to be one of those people. As the saying goes, "Sunshine is the best medicine."

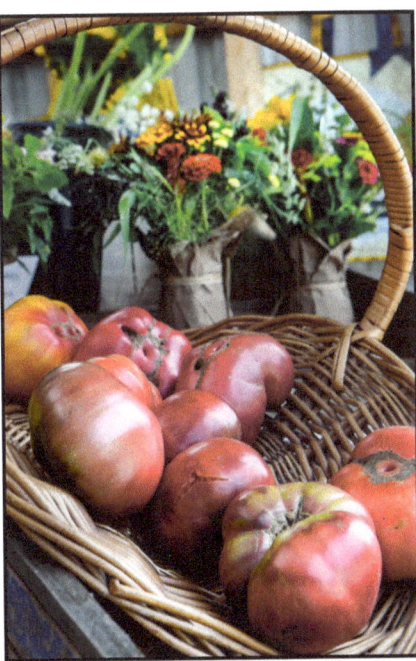
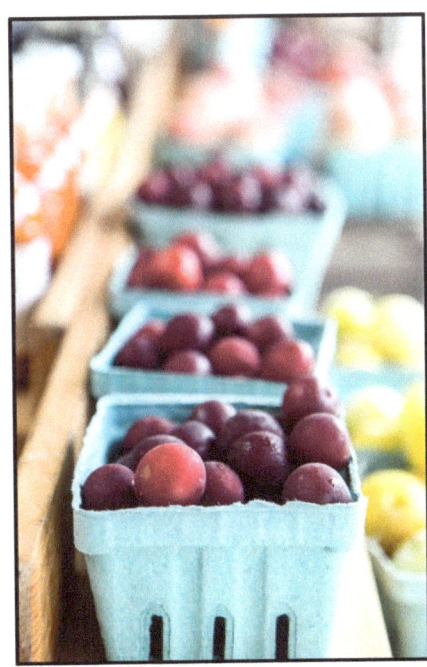

Farm to Table

Going right to the source of goodness

In the part of the country where I live, we are so blessed to be surrounded with an abundance of organic farms. Within a half-hour radius, you can drive through the most beautiful back roads and rolling hills sprinkled with farms. Mom and Pop farms offer CSA (Community Supported Agriculture) offerings and the Amish and Mennonite farms are known for their fresh raw dairy products, eggs, and vegetables. Farmer's markets pop up all over the place where you can purchase everything from local honey to freshly baked bread.

One of my favorite treats is to take a day to drive from farm to farm to purchase goodies. It's worth the trip to Jersey Hollow Farm outside of Kutztown, PA to buy eggs. They're so fresh that often times there's still a feather or two on them...I'm not kidding! Root vegetables are still covered in dirt, chickens roam free, and the cows

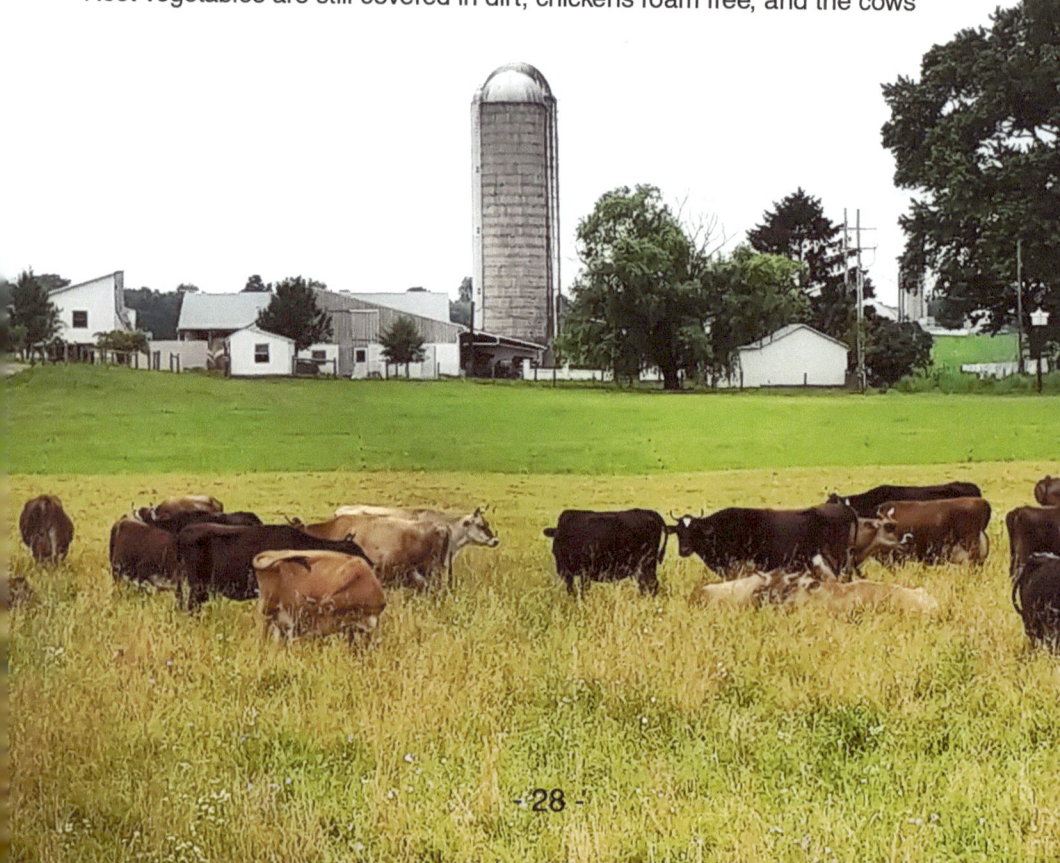

graze in the pasture. There's not a boxed product in site and you can actually talk to the people who grew the produce. It's heaven!

When the real world sets in with its long list of things to do, the luxury of a leisurely road trip is out of the question. That's where being part of a local CSA is so helpful. Each week I take home so many fresh vegetables that I might not otherwise buy at the grocery store. Eating what's in season is not only good for the body, but it forces us to be creative with recipes. I never made turnip soup until it was in the week's selection. I learned how to roast beets; and the things you can make with zucchini, well that's a book all in itself.

The other day I was making a quiche and was out of milk. So, I quickly ran into a nearby convenience-type gas station. As I walked in, it hit me in the face like a dazed kid in dodge ball. The amount of junk food lined up so pretty on the shelves was for too many people their reality of food. Not a fresh food item in sight. Is it any wonder why people's health is on the decline?

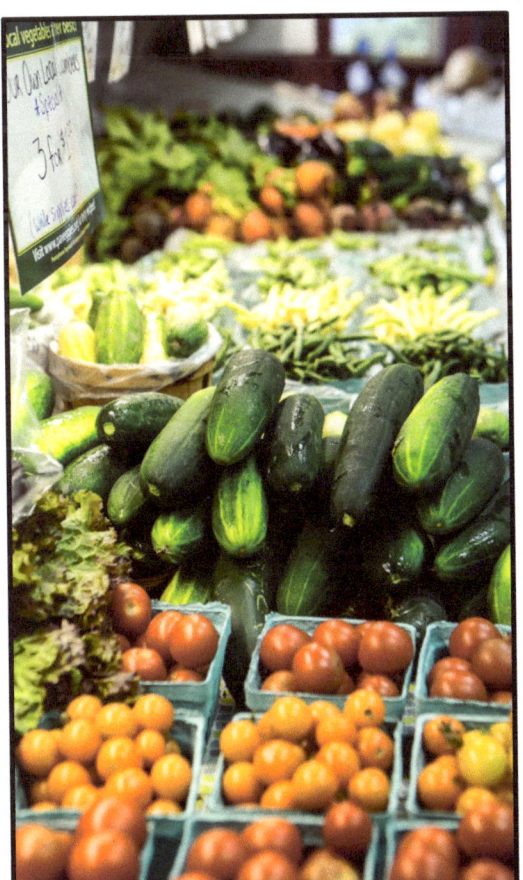

Yes, it's not always easy to take the time to hunt down fresh, organic fruits and vegetables, but your body will thank you for it. Go on an adventure, whether it's an hour or a whole day. The best part is that you can come home and eat it.

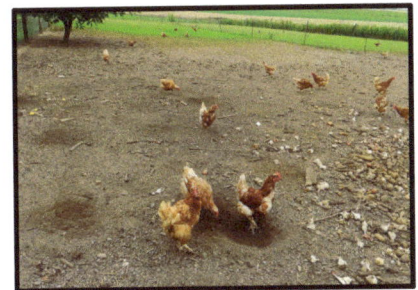

So Easy Vegetable Soup

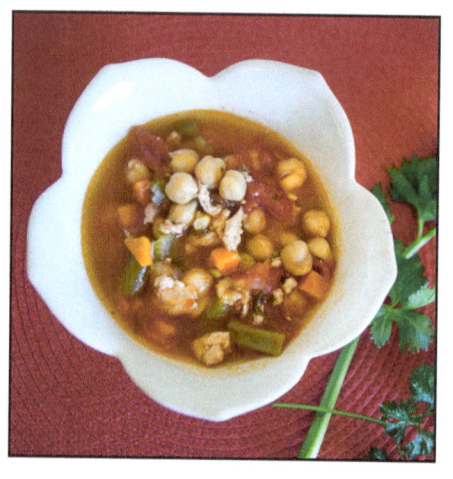

You're gonna need:

1/2 diced onion and 1 stalk celery
1/2 lb. ground chicken or turkey
one 14 oz. jar of whole tomatoes
32 oz. vegetable or chicken stock
1/2 of 16 oz. bag frozen mixed vegetables
one 15 oz. can of chickpeas, drained
fresh parsley sprig (or dried works too)
salt, pepper, dried oregano to taste

In a world where kids refuse to eat their vegetables, this soup is a savior for my grandson Logan. This picky little toddler refuses to eat most vegetables, but somehow, he loves my homemade soup. It's a sure way of getting vegetables into him. It's ridiculously easy to make, and you have full permission to experiment with any and all ingredients. I add either ground organic chicken or turkey for an extra protein punch, but vegetarians can easily leave that out. Sometimes I use chicken that was left over from a previous night's dinner and just dice it up really small. It's a great use of leftovers. I've also used both chicken and vegetable stock as well as bone broth as the base and had wonderful results with all three.

Although I have exact quantities for the ingredients, I want you to put in the amount you want. If you need a big pot of soup, then one pound of ground meat works well. Pour in as much of the frozen veggie bag as you want. Or if you are really industrious, chop your own fresh ones. On busy days, there's just not enough time to do that. Try sneaking in vegetables that are in season and see if anyone notices! Chickpeas are a wonderful addition for extra fiber and protein, but I've also used different types of beans. Although I'm not a big fan of adding extra carbs like pasta, feel free to add all kinds of tiny noodles or macaroni. Be daring! You can't really go wrong with this soup.

Here's what to do:

Sauté onions and celery in either ghee or avocado oil until tender. If you are using ground meat, add it to the onions and celery and cook until meat is done. Add the tomatoes and let simmer for a few minutes and then add the stock along with the frozen soup veggies and chickpeas. Cook for about 20 minutes. Add the chopped parsley leaves along with seasonings. Simmer for about 5 more minutes. Ladle out and enjoy a great lunch.

TIP: BOTH GHEE AND AVOCADO OIL HAVE A HIGH SMOKE POINT, SO IT'S A HEALTHIER OPTION.

I jar my own heirloom tomatoes every year; but if that's a crazy thought for you, store bought works just fine.

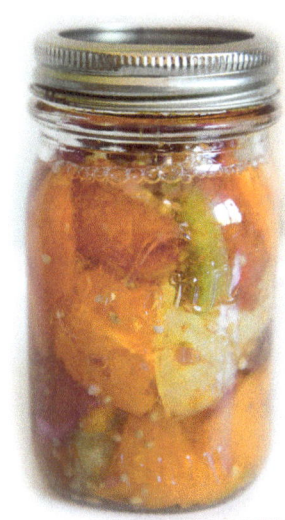

Food for Thought!

If you thought celery was just empty calories and a vehicle for peanut butter, think again. Celery has so many healing properties. It helps lower high cholesterol and inflammation, promotes liver health, boosts digestion, reduces bloating, and helps prevent urinary tract infections. Celery also contains a special type of ethanol extract that is useful in protecting the lining of the digestive tract from ulcers. Who knew! (peanut butter still tastes good on it, but almond butter is more delicious and it's much better for you.)

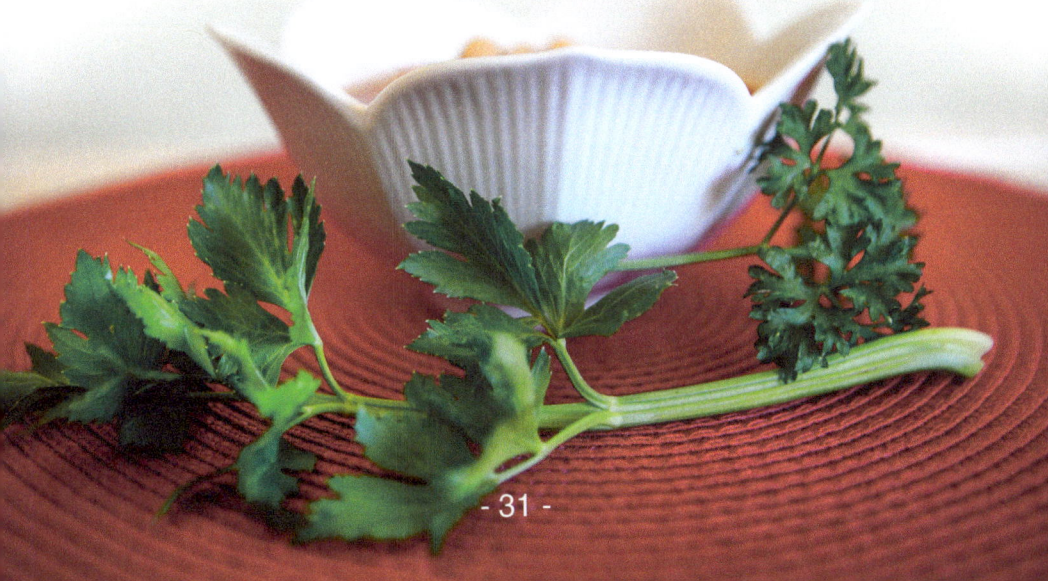

A Kitchen Garden

The healing properties of herbs

The most powerful health benefits of parsley include controlling cancer, managing diabetes, and rheumatoid arthritis, along with helping prevent osteoporosis. Parsley acts as a pain reliever with anti-inflammatory properties. It also provides relief from gastrointestinal issues such as bloating, indigestion, stomach cramps, and nausea. Parsley also helps strengthen the immune system.

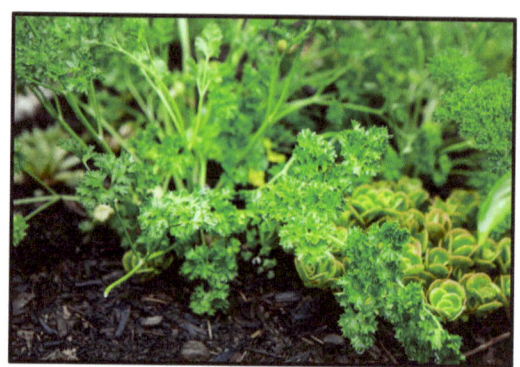

One of the most amazing ways to add both flavor and healing qualities to a dish is to add fresh herbs. You don't have to be a crazy gardener like I am to enjoy the benefits of freshly picked herbs. It just takes a flower pot filled with a few carefully selected plants to do the trick.

I love to sprinkle plants here and there in my perennial flower beds. Tuck a parsley plant here, a basil there, rosemary in between succulents, and before you know it, you have a kitchen garden. The go-to herbs in my garden are the ones that I cook with the most: rosemary, parsley, mint, and basil. Sage, curry, and thyme have also worked their way into the mix. The smell of these herbs is a treat to the senses. I can hardly walk past them without picking off a leaf, rubbing it between my fingers and taking a deep inhale. Heavenly!

Herbed Strawberries and Watermelon

A really simple way of amping up strawberries and watermelon is to add chopped basil and/or mint. Sprinkle crumbled feta cheese on top and drizzle a balsamic vinegar over the dish to finish it off, and you have a true summer treat. It's a two minute easy and delicious salad that packs a healing punch.

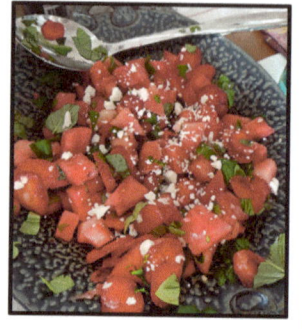

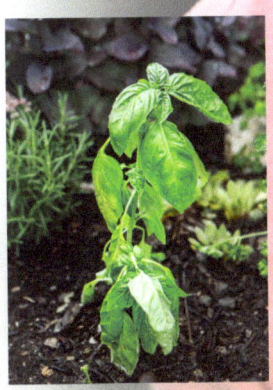

Basil is an excellent source of vitamin K and manganese; a very good source of copper, vitamin A (in the form of carotenoids such as beta-carotene), and vitamin C; and a good source of calcium, iron, folate, magnesium and omega-3 fatty acids. Did you know there are actually 35 different types of basil? Holy basil is the species of basil most known for its powerful healing qualities: anti-inflammatory, anti-bacterial and a powerful adaptogen, which helps the body to respond to stress.

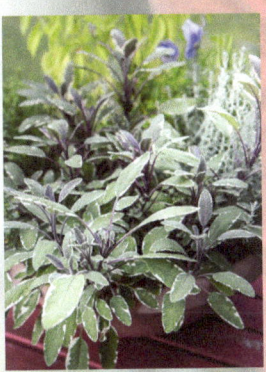

Sage is also an excellent source of fiber, vitamin A, folate, calcium, iron, magnesium, manganese, and B vitamins such as folic acid, thiamine, pyridoxine, and riboflavin in much higher doses than the recommended daily requirements, plus healthy amounts of vitamin C, vitamin E, thiamin, and copper. Pollinators like bees, hummingbirds, and butterflies can't resist the flowers of the sage plant; so having sage in your garden helps the pollination process.

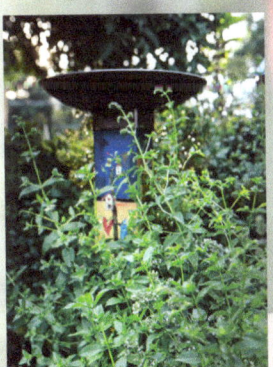

Mint is a great appetizer or palate cleanser. It also promotes digestion and soothes the stomach in case of indigestion or inflammation. When your stomach feels upset, drinking a cup of mint tea can give you relief. Mint contains phytonutrients with antioxidant-like properties, which may reduce cellular damage caused by oxidative stress. Did you know that 1/4 cup of spearmint provides nearly half of your daily needs of vitamin A?

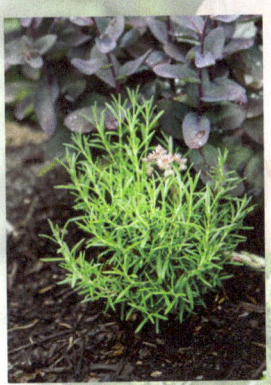

Rosemary was traditionally used to help alleviate muscle pain, improve memory, boost the immune and circulatory systems, and promote hair growth. Manganese, another of the more prominent minerals in rosemary, plays a critical antioxidant role in the body. Rosemary, when used regularly, can actively protect the lungs by preventing fluid accumulation and help to remove phlegm and excess mucus that blocks the respiratory tract.

The Perfect Duo

Tomato soup and grilled cheese!

Nothing goes better with tomato soup than a grilled cheese sandwich. This grilled cheese gets kicked up a thousand times to become an ooey gooey decadent panini that makes your mouth water. It brings back all your childhood memories, but with all the sophistication of adult indulgence.

Picture this: start with a fresh organic sourdough bread sliced thick. Butter each slice so it will sizzle on the panini maker. For the inside of the panini, start by spreading a thin layer of ricotta cheese on one slice of bread, layer fresh mozzarella and a creamy slice of brie on top of the ricotta. These three cheeses will melt together beautifully. Now get creative! Drizzle honey over the cheese and spread a gourmet jam on the second slice. I love the Stonewall Kitchen brand. Experiment with Fig & Walnut Butter, Bourbon Bacon Jam, or Bourbon Pear Onion Jam. Use your imagination. You can also use sliced dried figs instead of jam. There are endless combinations of goodness possible. Be prepared to leave out a giant moan on the first bite.

Tomatoes are a rich source of lycopene, beta-carotene, folate, potassium, vitamin C, flavonoids, and vitamin E that may protect lipoproteins and vascular cells from oxidation, which is what causes plaque to build up in your arteries. Even though tomatoes have lots of benefits, they are in the nightshade family. If you have any inflammation in your body, then nightshades are not the best thing to eat. Be careful!

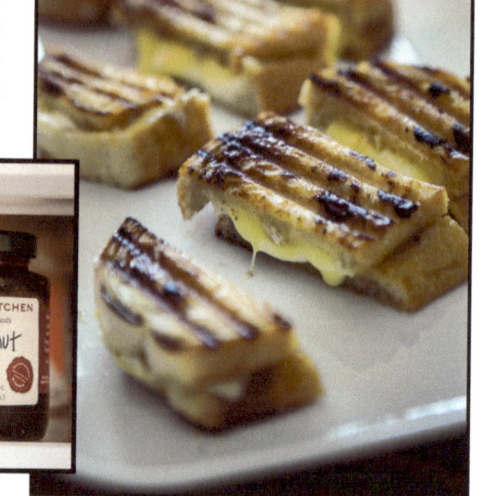

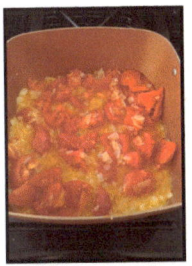
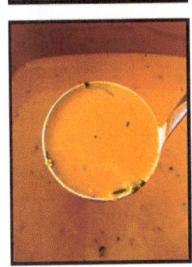
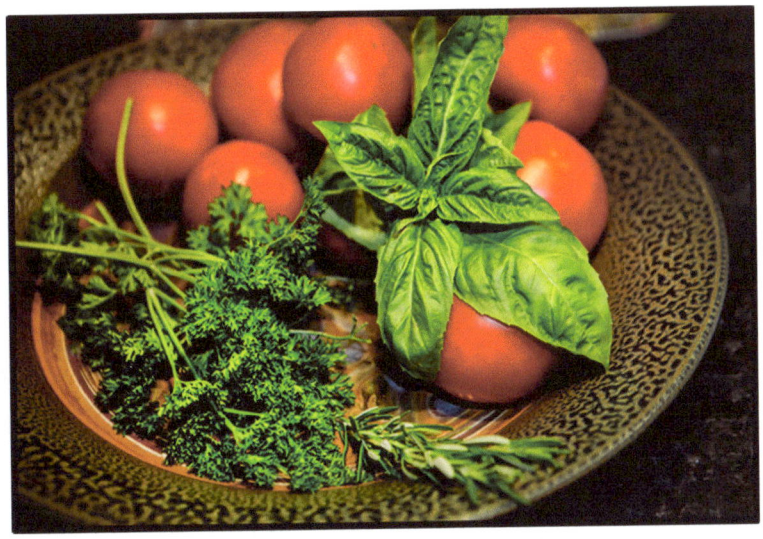

You're gonna need:

1 medium white or yellow onion; 1 clove chopped garlic; 6 tablespoons (3/4 stick) butter; two 14.5 ounce cans diced tomatoes or about 5 ripe whole tomatoes peeled and cut into chunks; one 46 ounce bottle or can tomato juice; 3 tablespoons sugar; 1 vegetable bouillon cube; 1/4 tsp. Noga N.17 spice, optional (bought from laboiteny.com) Freshly ground black pepper and salt to taste; 1 1/2 cups heavy cream; 1/4 cup chopped fresh basil; 1/4 cup chopped parsley.

Here's what to do:

This is NOT the tomato soup in a can that we all grew up on! It's fresh, delicious and sooooooooo summery. The fresher the tomatoes, the better this soup is going to taste. I suggest making it when tomatoes are in season, right from the garden or farmer's market.

To begin, dice the onion and the garlic. Melt the butter in a large pot. Toss in the onion and garlic and cook until translucent. Stir in the diced tomatoes and give the tomatoes a chance to meet and greet the onions for a few minutes. Pour in the tomato juice.

In order to counter the acidity of the tomatoes, add 3 tablespoons of sugar. Some tomatoes and juice have more of an acidic bite than others, so you can play with the amount of sugar to add. Next, add 1 vegetable bouillon cube along with the Noga N.17 spice and salt and pepper. Simmer for about 15 minutes. This is the perfect time to have a sip of wine and enjoy the moment.

I love using an immersion blender to puree soup. Puree the soup until it is almost smooth, leaving tiny bits here and there. Stir in the heavy cream. Top with the chopped basil and parsley. You are ready to dip that panini in your soup!

Creating Sacred Space

Into every vase a few weeds should fall

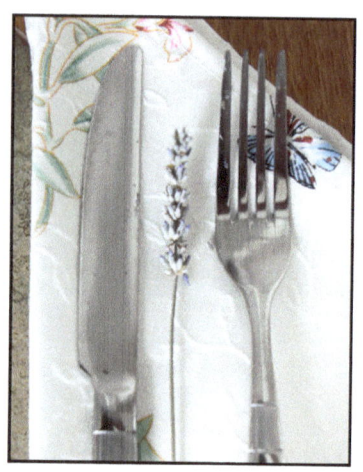

Just a sprig of lavendar mixed in with your place settings makes all the difference.

If you are lucky enough to have a garden, and I have 27 of them (I know I'm a bit crazy), then you have the opportunity to create beauty and serenity in your life. I'm far from a floral designer, but I followed my dear yoga teacher Erin's example of how to mix and match the simplest things together to create beauty. I'd come into yoga class and there would be one flower or a little sprig of something in a tiny glass container set upon a scarf. It was so simple, and yet it was so beautiful. Why didn't I think of that! Now I do.

As life gets busier and busier, being outside in nature "feeds" our soul. I love to wander around my yard and look for the not-so-obvious choices. The loner dandelion, the twig of leftover asparagus, the weed that everyone pulls out of their yard, the rogue daisy or overzealous mint that wants to take over the world are all enthusiastic volunteers just waiting to be picked.

So... no vases, you say? Think outside the box and look inside your cabinets. I found a cute little creamer that I rarely use, and it became the perfect vase for a handful of freshly picked flowers. If you don't have a flower garden, it's not a problem. Just pick some up when you go grocery shopping. It's the thought that counts. Taking care of ourselves is more than putting good food in our mouth. It's about feeding our soul as well. We can eat all the organic produce we can find, but if our soul isn't also nourished, the odds are that we probably won't be healthy. The ritual of picking flowers is as important as picking fresh vegetables. Go out, be bold, pick that weed!

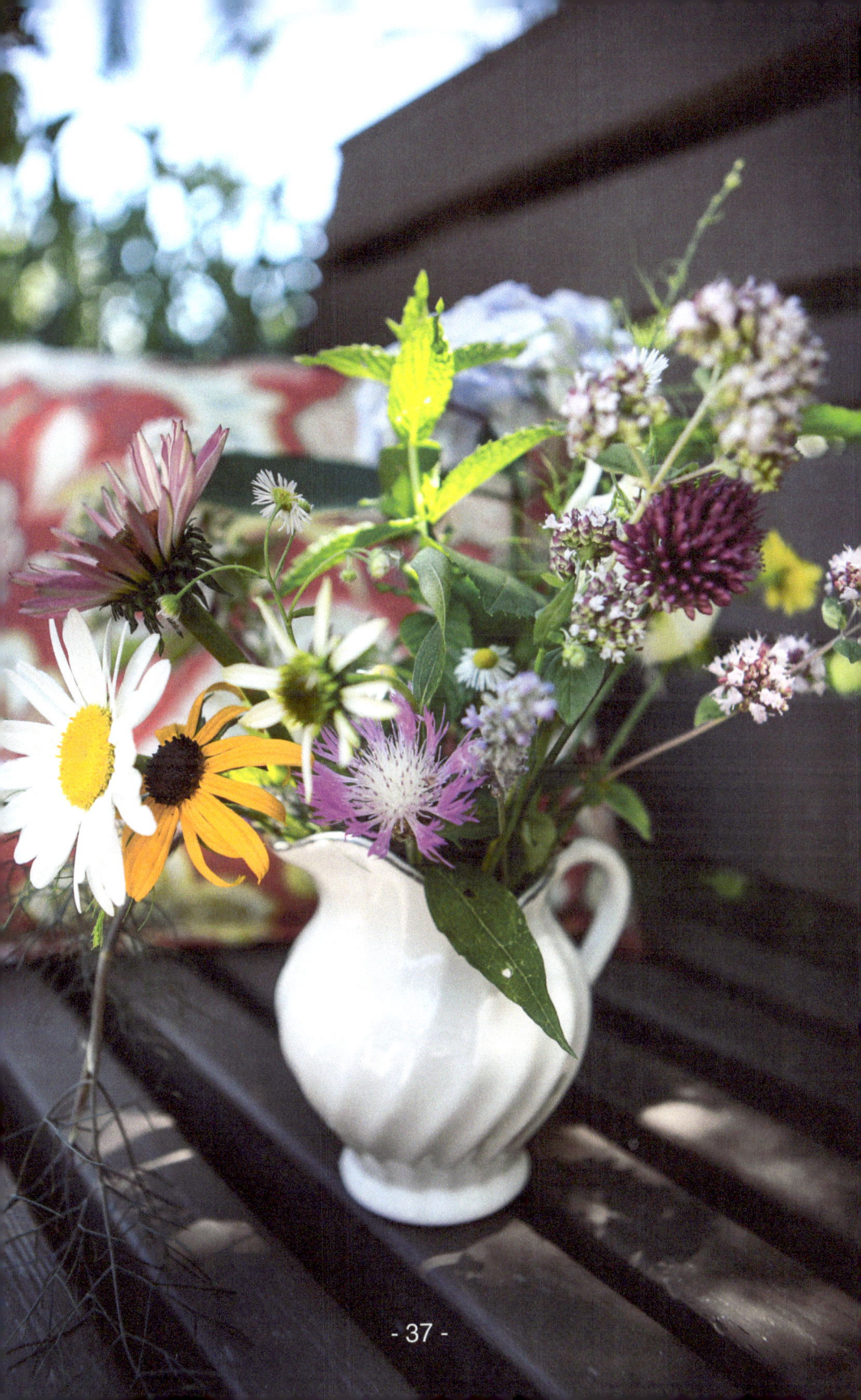

Summery Zucchini Soup

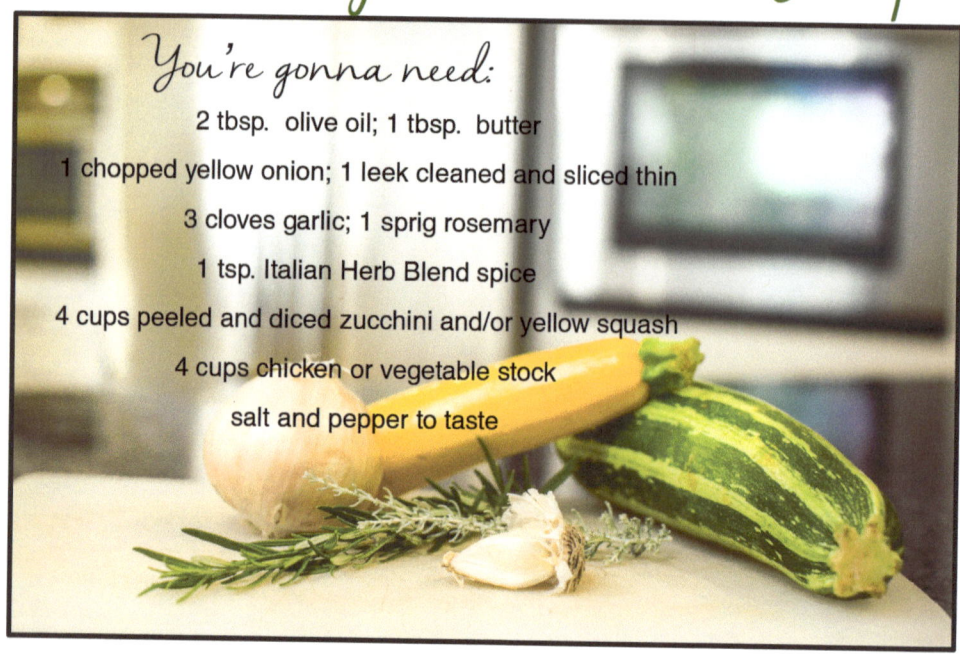

You're gonna need:

2 tbsp. olive oil; 1 tbsp. butter

1 chopped yellow onion; 1 leek cleaned and sliced thin

3 cloves garlic; 1 sprig rosemary

1 tsp. Italian Herb Blend spice

4 cups peeled and diced zucchini and/or yellow squash

4 cups chicken or vegetable stock

salt and pepper to taste

Here's what to do:

First: Smash and dice your garlic and set it aside. Any time there is garlic in a recipe, you should chop it first. The longer the garlic sits, the more chance it has to retain its healing properties. So no matter where in a recipe it calls for garlic to be added, always smash and dice it as the first thing you do.

Heat the olive oil and butter in a soup pot. Add the chopped onion and leek (make sure you have cleaned the leek thoroughly and sliced it into thin slivers, discarding most of the green leaves at the top of the leek) and simmer until translucent.

Chop the rosemary into tiny bits and stir it into the pot along with your garlic and the teaspoon of Italian Herb Blend. Cook 3 to 5 minutes. This is a great time to just stop, take a deep breath, and soak in the amazing smell of simmering rosemary.

Add the chopped zucchini and squash. Simmer for about 5 more minutes. This will allow the zucchini to really soak up all the goodness of the rosemary. Pour in the stock and then salt and pepper to taste. Cover and simmer until zucchini are soft and tender (about 25 minutes).

Using an immersion blender, puree soup until smooth and creamy. Pour soup into your favorite bowl and enjoy the freshness that summer offers.

Garlic contains so many antibiotic and antibacterial properties. Crushing garlic releases the allicin within the bulb, which is the nutrient that is thought to contain the most potent form of antibiotic material in garlic.

The more the garlic is crushed and smashed, the more potent allicin is released. Many scientists suggest chopping or dicing your garlic, then letting it stand for ten minutes to let the alliinase do its work and form as much allicin as possible before it's neutralized by heat.

It turns out that heat neutralizes the health-giving benefits of allicin! So, the next time you're cooking, be sure to mince your garlic first thing, then let it stand. By the time you're done getting the rest of your ingredients ready, those crushed cloves will have a lot of allicin moving around in their cells.

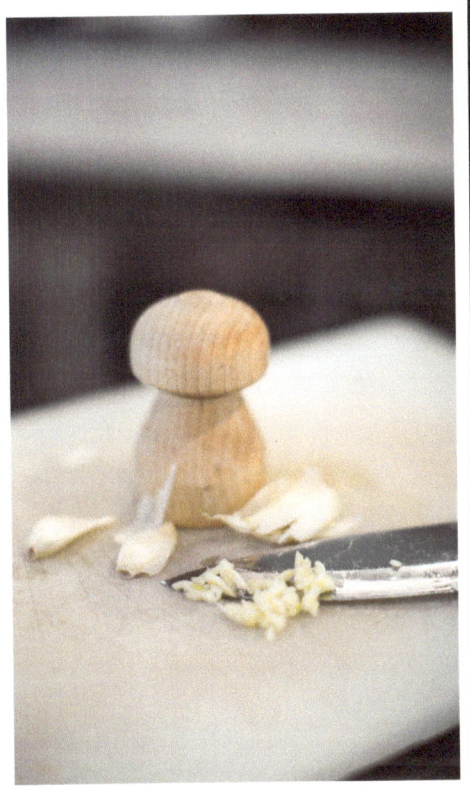

Food for Thought!

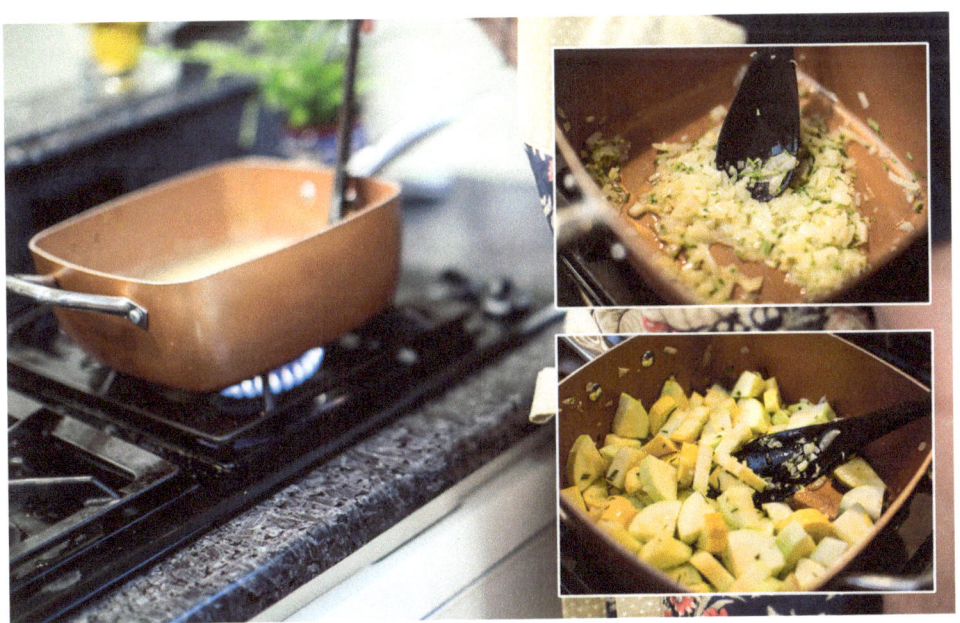

Home Sweet Home

Ways to create a haven from the storm

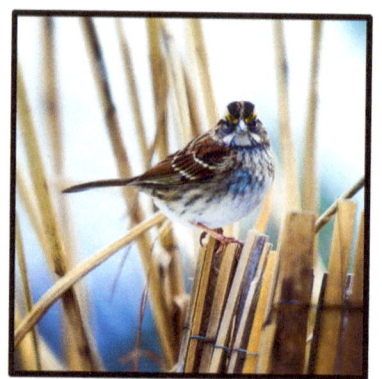

A tiny bird peeks its head out of the birdhouse. It looks around to see if it's safe to take flight and leave the nest. It's a crazy world out there, full of all kinds of perils..... there might be a cat lurking in the grass just waiting for an easy lunch; but in the nest it's warm, cozy, and safe. There are times when I watch this little bird outside my kitchen window for hours. In and out, in and out, until I lose count of the trips to who knows where. It makes me wonder about life and the craziness we all go through on any given day. We rush here and there with a jam-packed schedule. There's so much to do and so little time to do it, but each time we come back home.

If we are lucky, our home is a place of refuge, much like the nest is to this bird. It should be our safe haven when so many things in the world seem so out of control. I'm no Martha Stewart, although my sisters tell me I am, but I choose to surround myself in serenity as much as possible. I've been taught that the food we put in our mouth is only secondary to what really feeds us. Our relationships, career, spirituality, and our physical activity, along with our home environment, all play a major role in our total health. It's so important to have balance in all of these areas.

Sometimes it's the littlest things that make the biggest impact. There are things we can all do, regardless of where we live or how much money we have, to "feed" our soul and calm our mind. You can turn up the music, light a candle, open a window on a nice day, put out a pretty place mat for dinner, and surround yourself with pictures of family and friends. You know what to do. As the saying goes, "Home truly is where the heart is", so let's all make our nest just a little sweeter.

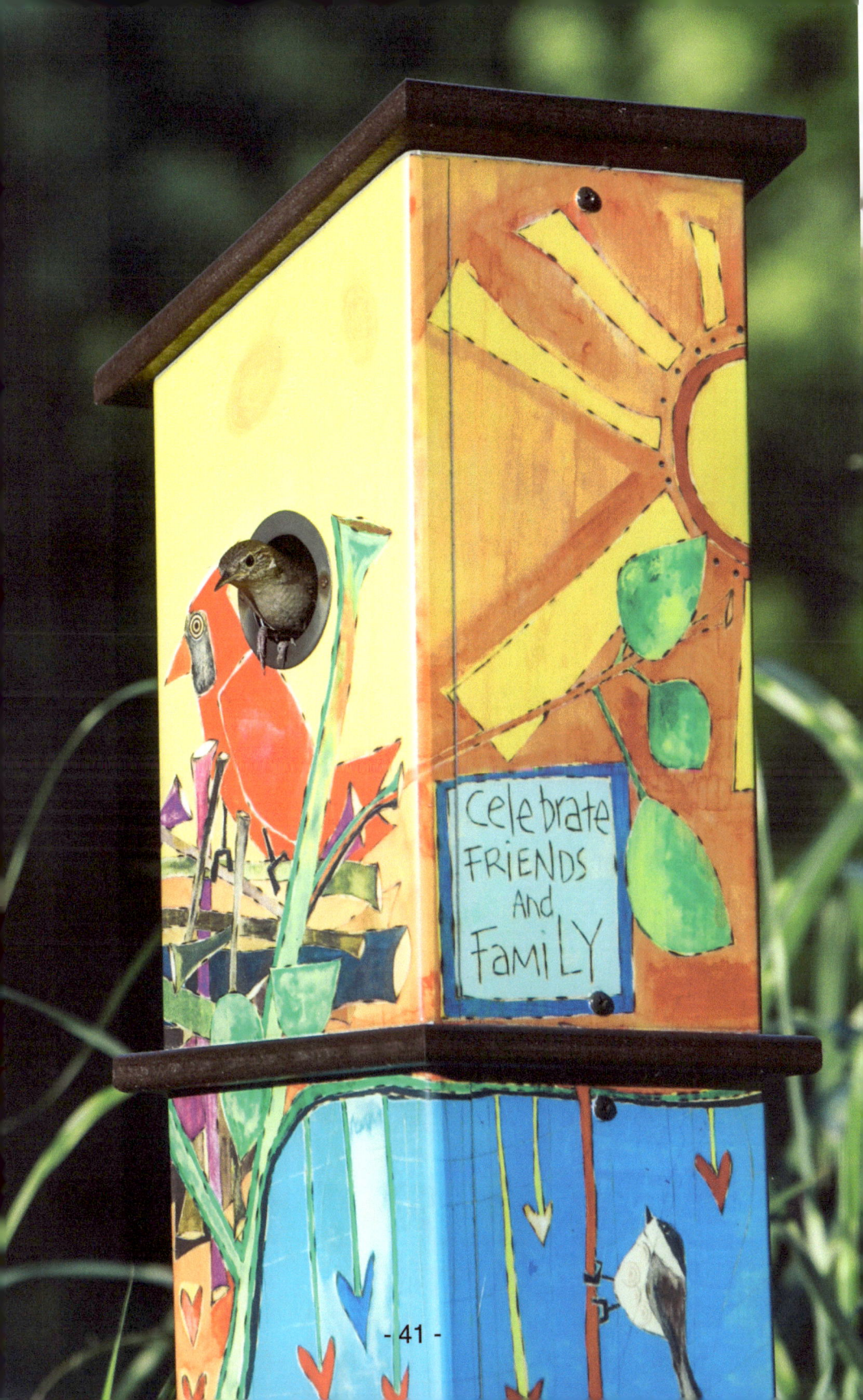

About Miso

Miso paste is an Asian seasoning made by fermenting a mixture of soybeans, barley, brown rice, and several other grains with a fungus, Aspergillus oryzae. The result of this fermentation is a smooth textured paste with a strong, salty flavor. Often used in Asian cooking, miso is a healthy, probiotic food that helps support digestion by adding beneficial microorganisms to your digestive tract.

Probiotic foods like miso paste have a number of health benefits. In addition to contributing new bacteria to your existing intestinal colonies, miso can also help you overcome intestinal illness, including diarrhea.

An easy way to incorporate miso into your diet is to simply add a spoonful of miso to oil and vinegar and use it as a salad dressing. Your digestive tract will thank you for it; and it's easy, healthy, and tasty.

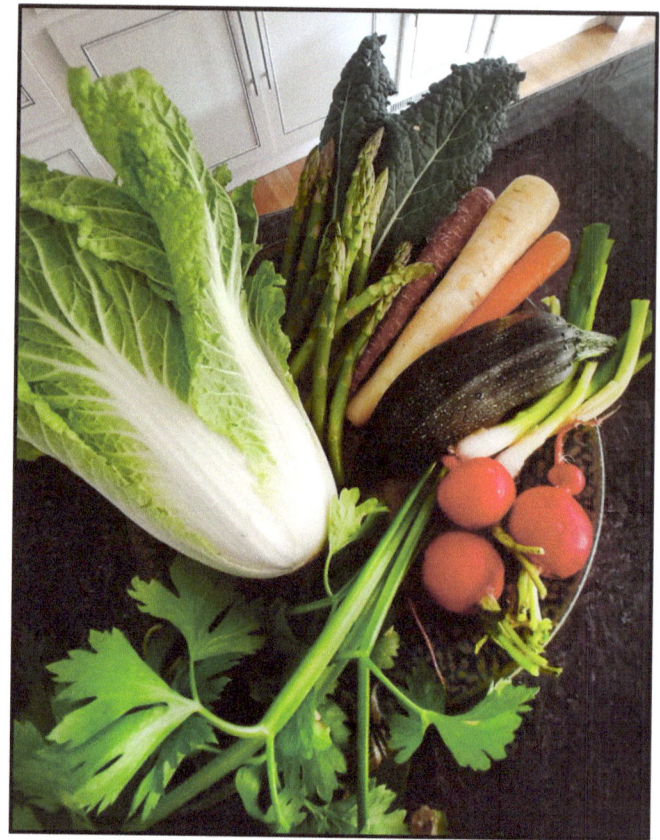

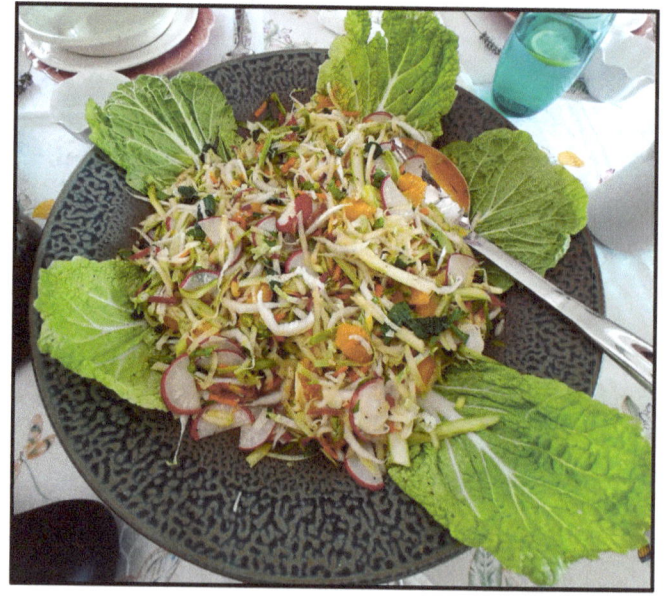

Fresh Summer Slaw

The bounty of summer vegetables is endless. Trying to use them all before they go bad can be a full-time job, unless you use them all in this super fresh and crunchy slaw. I was inspired by a recipe in one of my favorite cookbooks, "The First Mess" for this recipe. Use all kinds of chopping styles: shred some, shave some, dice or slice others, and use a veggie noodle spiralizer for the zucchini. Go crazy!

You're gonna need:

Zucchini, asparagus spears, kale leaves, carrots, celery stalks, napa cabbage, green onions, radishes, celery.

Here's what to do:

1. After using an assortment of cutting methods to make this salad look pretty, mix all the veggies together and season with salt and pepper. Use napa cabbage leaves to decorate the plate before spooning the veggie mix on top.

2. Pour miso dressing over the salad and sprinkle chia seeds on top.

3. Optional yummies could include using Mandarin oranges or mangos to top off the salad.

CITRUS MISO DRESSING INGREDIENTS

1/4 cup juice of a freshly squeezed orange
1 tablespoon fresh lime juice
1 garlic clove, finely chopped
2 teaspoons light chickpea miso
1/4 teaspoon gluten-free tamari soy sauce
1/4 teaspoon Dijon mustard
1/4 cup olive oil
1 tsp. honey
ground black pepper

Mix the above ingredients in a glass jar. Shake well or use an immersion blender until smooth. Add a little water if the dressing is too thick.

Par for the Course

Take advantage of the "do-overs" in life

Awwww.... golf. You either love it or hate it. It's been quite a few years since I'd swung a club, but I had the chance to enjoy a day out with some ladies for a friendly, no-pressure nine holes. Talk about tapping into some good old muscle memory!

What I forgot that I knew was that the game of golf has so many analogies to the game of life. For example, you step up to the tee. You think you have everything lined up perfectly. In your mind's eye you see the ball sailing through the air and landing at just the right spot so you have a great second shot position. It has to work; after all, you envisioned it perfectly, therefore it will happen. Wrong! You either top the ball, hit it into the rough, aim in the entirely wrong direction, or land in a sand trap. Oh well, another day at the beach as they say. With lots of encouragement from teammates and a little humility from yourself, you announce that you want "a do-over". A Mulligan, to be exact. Most times, the second shot is so much better. I said most times, but not always. We either enthusiastically move to the next shot happy that we did a better job or we sulk our way to where the ball disappointingly landed.

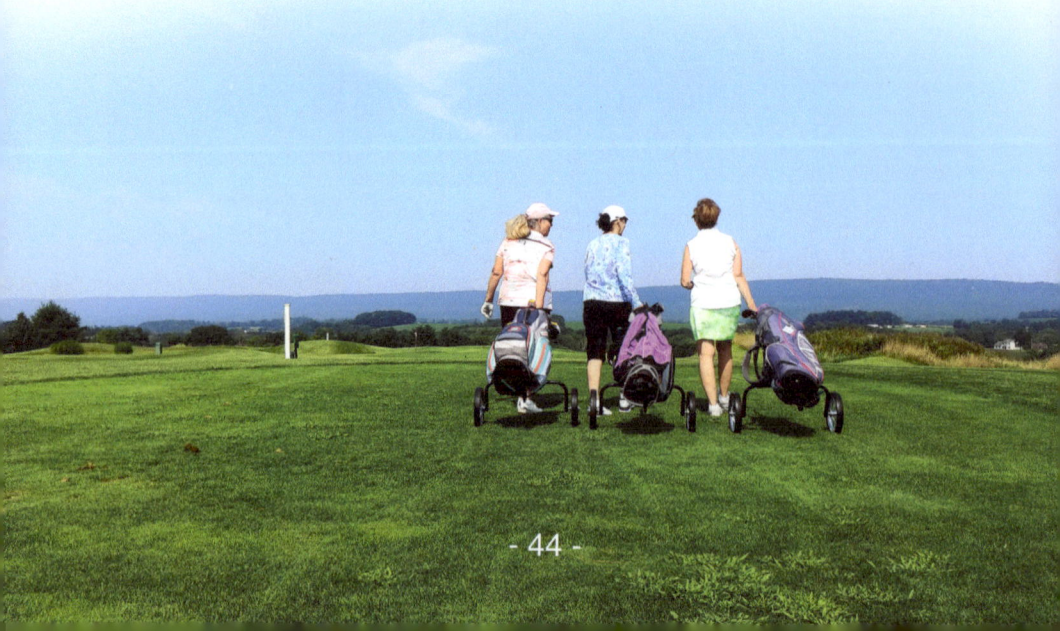

Life is like that in so many ways. We make a plan. We see the goal with crystal clear vision. We think we have everything lined up perfectly. We expect it to work out because that's what should happen. Once again, wrong! So many of life's lessons are learned by trial and error. How many do-overs does it take for our efforts to pay off? I guess as many as it takes. And this is where the frustration sets in. We can either throw our clubs to the ground, say a few cuss words and vow to give up completely, or we can just pick up the ball and move to the next tee. That's what we have to do in life, too. We land in the wrong situation, we pick ourselves up, dust ourselves off, and move on to another day in the hopes that tomorrow will be better.

Like golf, life is a game where we put so much pressure on ourselves to measure up to a certain standard. The hole is marked a par three. What if I don't get there in three...what if it takes six swings to finally get it in the hole? How many times do I really have to hit out of the rough!!!! Why can't I just land on the fairway for once. It's so much easier to make the shot from such a nice smooth surface. Think about how many of our life's challenges come from the rough. Rarely is it smooth sailing for long before we land in the rough again. But that's life. They always say, and I've always been curious as to exactly who "they" are, that we grow the most from challenges and not from the times of smooth sailing. Knowing this doesn't make it any easier.

It was a great day out on the course. A clear, sunny day after days and days of rain. The views were stunning. The conversations between the ladies was uplifting and gratifying. In the end, it didn't matter how many shots it took to get in the hole. In fact, we didn't even keep score. Making par wasn't important. We squealed like school girls when we hit a great shot and kept going when we didn't.

And so it goes with life. We can either fill our days with keeping score and worrying about each and every shot we take in life, or we can just enjoy everything else that happens in our life that gives us joy. Life is about friendship, seeing the beauty in a sunny day, and relaxing into the moment even when life's ball is in the rough. Go ahead, pick up the ball and put it on the fairway. Don't even care if someone's looking. Take the do-over.

Facing the Storm

What's Eating You

Just Breathe

The Perfect Recipe

Autumn

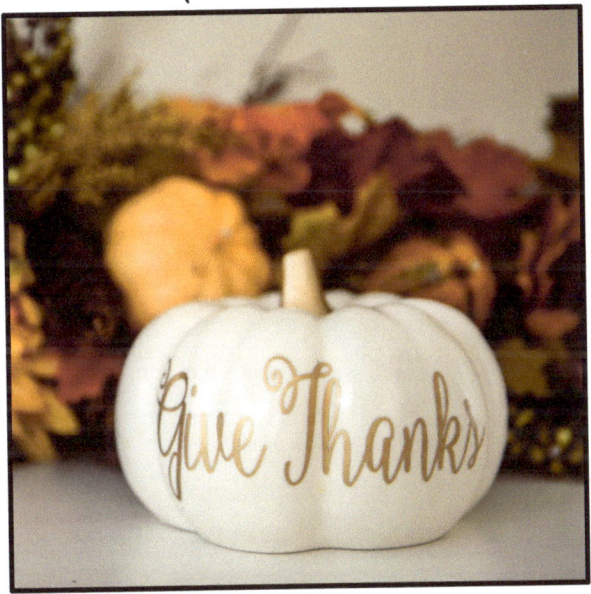

Fall into a state of gratitude

A Season of Change

Basking in the golden glow of fall

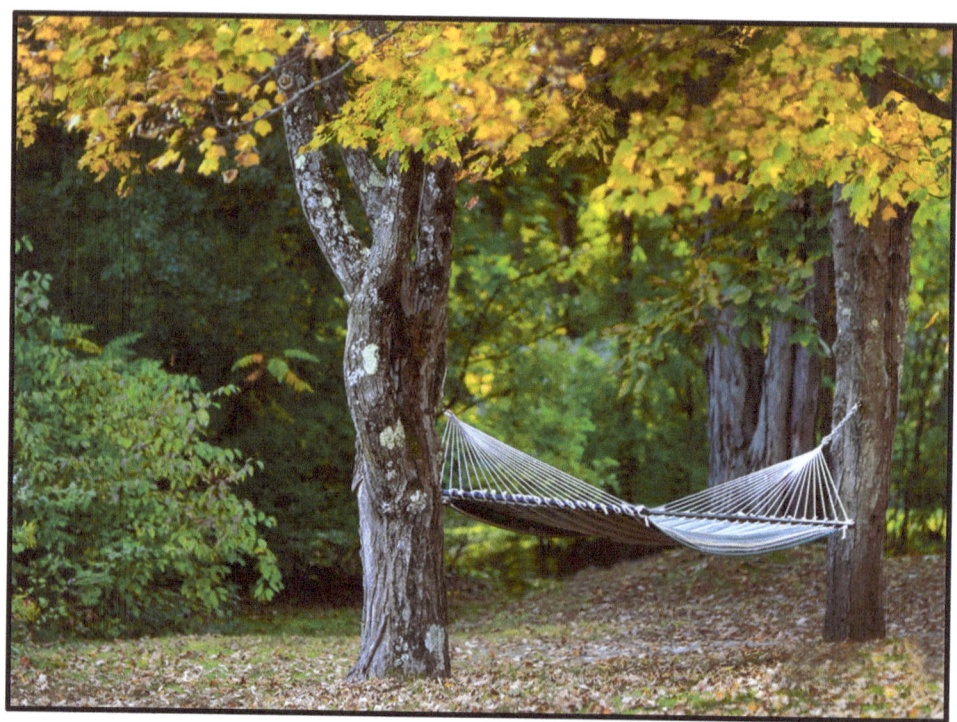

Fall! One of the most beautiful times of year. Humid hot days are traded for crisp cool nights. Trees get to show off their full potential in a blaze of red, yellow, and orange. Pumpkin spice takes over everything! We say goodbye to flip flops and look forward to wearing leggings and boots. There's only one thing wrong with fall: winter follows. The very fact that the warm golden days of autumn are followed by the bleak dreary days of an icy cold winter, challenges us to be really present to the moment. I personally struggle with thoughts of, "Oh no; it's almost winter", when in reality it's months away. Talk about nature's perfect challenge to our state of mind: each time my mind goes to that "oh no" place, I have to remind myself to focus on what is, and not what's in the future. At that point, all we can really do is stop and say, "Wow, what a beautiful day it is today! Right now, at this moment, it's awesome."

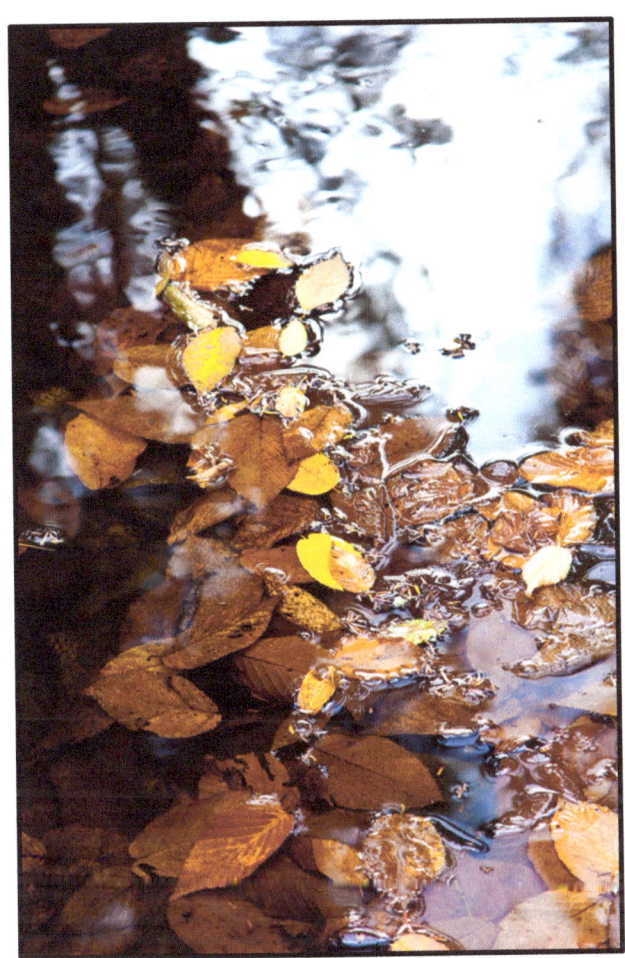

> "Autum is a second spring where every leaf is a flower."
>
> Albert Camus

    If we think about the four seasons as a symbolic representation of our lives, and if we happen to be in the fall of our life, that means that we have a lot to do before winter. This is the time to, as they say, "Give it hell". It's a time to let our true colors show and enjoy flaunting them in their fullest glory. Maybe there are days when we wake up stiff, and maybe we can't do the same things we used to do with as much intensity as before; but, nevertheless, we can still take the proverbial bull by the horns and teach it a thing or two. For those of us in the fall of our lives, we bring with it two seasons of experience and knowledge. To me, using those tools to the fullest is like the trees who change their leaves from a pretty but safe green to an outrageous display of color. I don't know about you, but I'm gonna live the fall of my life with all the color and intensity that I can.

Facing the Storm

Calming the mind in the midst of uncertainty

Sometimes you just have to weed the garden with thunder in the background. You have to be willing to go out there, yank out some troublesome weeds or clear an overgrown path even though you know the storm is coming. It would be ridiculous to do it while it's lightning, but with thunder in the background, maybe not so much. Life is like that. Gardening is a metaphor for life. It's the time where I can just pull weeds and think about life; it's a working meditation. People often say, "Oh, I could never meditate. I can't sit still long enough." You don't really have to sit still to connect to your inner voice. Sometimes you could just wash dishes or iron, but very few people iron anymore. If you're a gardener, you could pull weeds. Lots of people do that. I do that. I love doing that. It's in those moments when I let my mind run free that I think about life: what I've done, what it's done to me, where I've been, and where I might be going.

I know that the sum of these 67 years is an accumulation of the good, the bad, and sometimes the ugly; but life always works out for the best even when we are certain it hasn't. No matter what I've been through, it just made me stronger. For me, it made my faith deeper. It gave me a sense of purpose and hope. It's a true test of faith in divine timing to never quite know what's around the corner. There are times when I'm momentarily freaking out, but everyone deserves a good freak out every now and again. That's just being human.

We all know that you have to protect yourself in life, but in gardening there are a few precautions you have to take, too. Always wear gloves so the stickers seem less ouchy. Never pull poison with your bare hands, it will itch like hell the next day. If you don't disturb the bees, they won't bother you. Sometimes you have to cut plants down halfway just to see them come back twice as full and more beautiful than before you cut them.

Life's like that. Sometimes we get nipped in the bud; but if we keep trying, we're going to come back twice as strong and more beautiful than ever. Don't be afraid of a little thunder in your life. A rainbow just might be in your future.

My heart is in the garden. Gardening is a matter of your enthusiasm holding up until your back gets used to it. How deeply seated in the human heart is the liking for gardens. Everything that slows us down and forces patience; everything that sets us back into the slow circles of nature is a help. Garden as though you will live forever. Learn to be an observer in all seasons. The greatest gift of the garden is the restoration of the five senses.

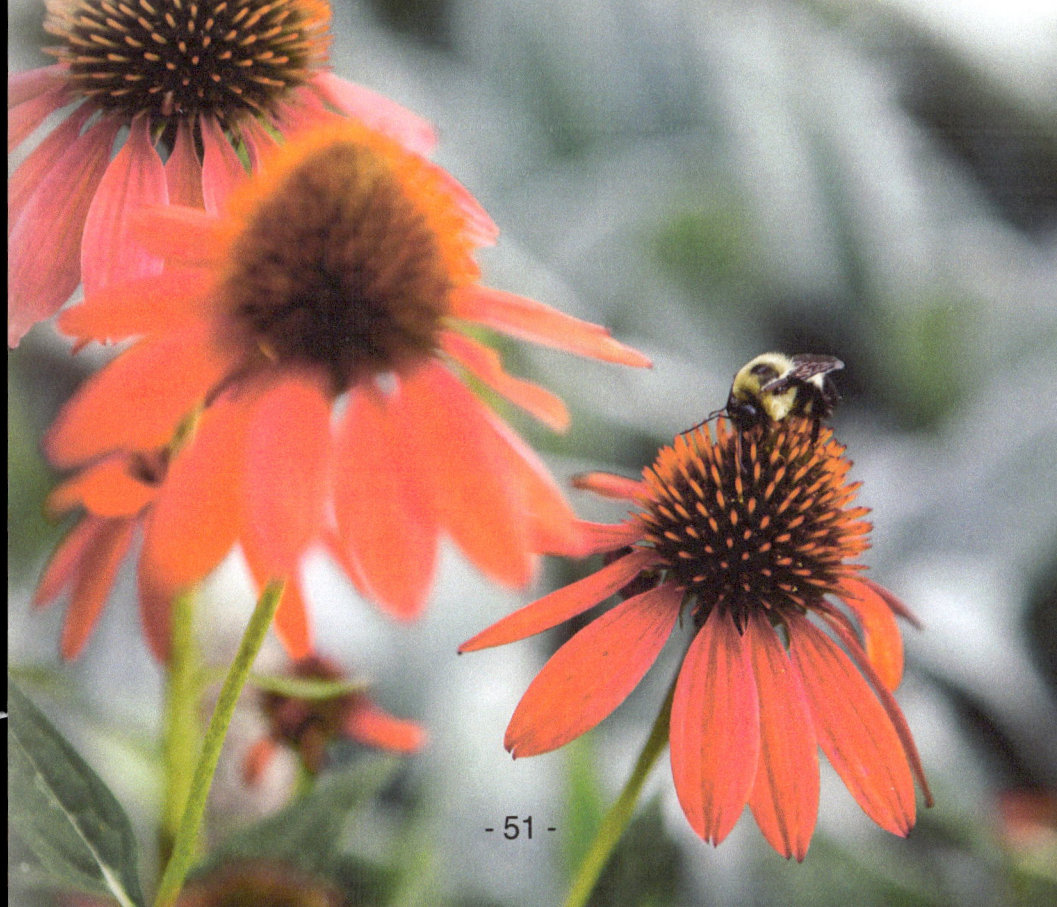

Empty the Fridge Quiche

Yes, real men will eat this quiche! This recipe is so easy; and the quiche will last several days in the refrigerator, making it another quick grab-n-go option when you are short on time or just not in the mood to cook. Sometimes it's breakfast, other times a lunch, and at dinner it goes great with a salad or soup. The combination of ingredients is only limited by your imagination and what's in your fridge. I rarely make the exact same quiche twice. However, every quiche starts with the same basic ingredients.

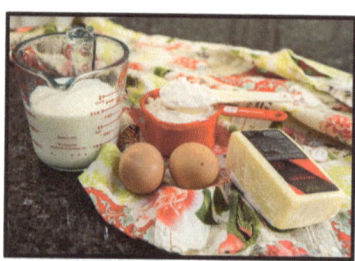

BASIC STARTER INGREDIENTS: 2 eggs; 1 cup plus 1 tbsp. flour; 1 tsp. salt; 1/8 tsp. pepper; 1 1/2 cups milk; 6 to 8 oz. grated cheese.

Here's what to do:

I've used both regular flour and gluten free flour for this recipe with good results. For the type of cheese, you just need a good cheese that melts easy. Options are American, Cheddar, Monterey Jack, Colby, Swiss, and my favorite, Havarti. I've often used a combination of types just to use up random cheeses that I have on hand. This quiche, unfortunately, is not a good option for vegans or for those people who have issues with dairy.

Start by combining all the starter ingredients in a large mixing bowl and set aside.

Another ingredient I always use is sautéed onions. I think it adds so much flavor. Typically, about 1/2 onion does the trick. (if you don't like onions, you can leave them out.)

I usually mix and match at least two or three other ingredients to add to the batter.

CHOOSE FROM:
Broccoli, tomatoes, bacon, ham, turkey, asparagus, spinach, sun dried tomatoes, zucchini, mushrooms, peppers. If I am using bacon, I prepare it separately, let it cool and then crumble it up. I do the same with mushrooms. I sauté them in butter until they are nice and golden brown. I never add them raw to the mix. Spinach is another ingredient that works better if sautéed first and then added.

Pour your quiche into a greased and floured quiche dish and then garnish with sliced tomatoes on top and sprinkle with either seasoned salt or Emeril's Essence seasoning.

Bake at 400 degrees for 25 minutes. This crustless quiche will rise up and look as beautiful as it is delicious.

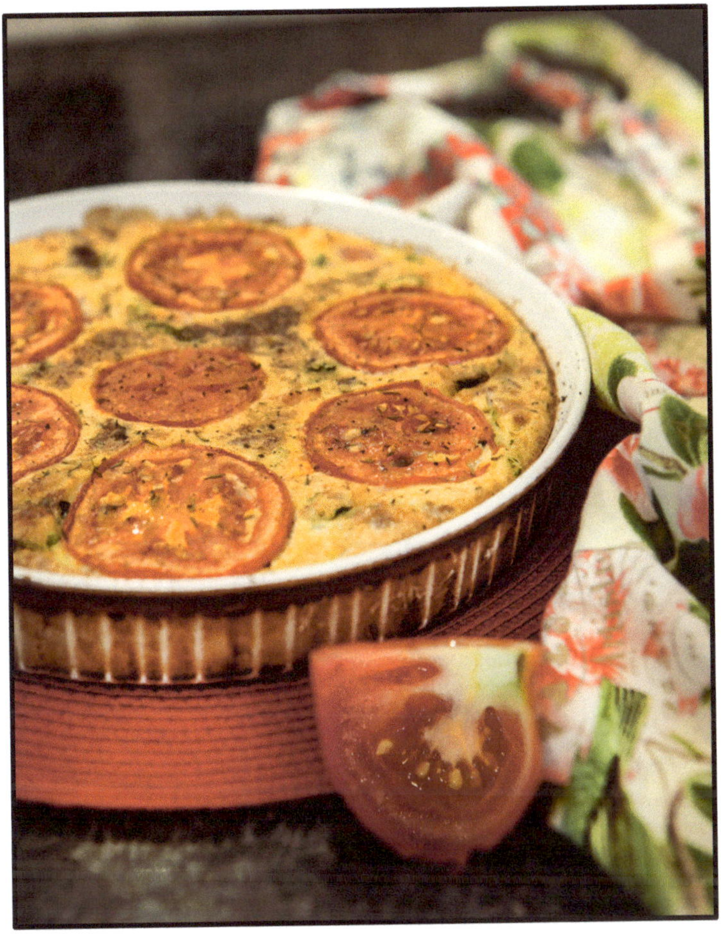

Food for Thought!

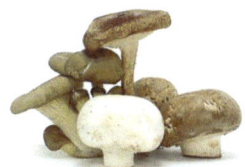

Cremini mushrooms are among the only natural food sources of vitamin D. And mushrooms are one of the few foods that contain a trace mineral that helps your body use oxygen efficiently.

Mushrooms are a good source of selenium, an antioxidant mineral, as well as copper, niacin, potassium and phosphorous. Mushrooms are also a source of protein, vitamin C and iron. Because mushroom's cell walls are indigestible unless exposed to heat, you must cook mushrooms to get their nutritional benefits. Mushrooms also help alkalize the body, which has a connection to improved immunity. A balanced pH level is crucial to health because disease cannot grow in an alkaline environment. Eating more mushrooms is also one way to lower cholesterol levels naturally. Many types of mushrooms help lower LDL or "bad" cholesterol and keeps arteries from hardening, which are risk factors for heart disease.

What's Eating You

Uncovering the root of cravings

You know when someone notices a mood you're in or how you might be acting, and says, "What's eating at you?" Funny how the word "eating" is used to describe something that might not even have anything to do with food. It could be a work-related issue, a fight you had with a family member, or simply stress from the world we live in. The reality is that often times what we put in our mouth is directly related to what's eating us. When we are super happy or busy doing something we love, actual food might be the last thing on our minds. However, let something really upset us and there's no telling how much ice cream we might eat!

What's also interesting about food cravings is that an urge you might have today could actually be triggered by a past memory of a childhood food and the related emotions that surround it. Sometimes that food comforted you, like tea and "jelly toast" when you had a belly ache and your mom just wanted you to feel better. Think about it. The cravings we have today have a direct link to experiences from our past. That's why when we are ready to fall off the wagon with a food we know we shouldn't eat, it might be best to stop and think about why we want to eat that food. It's called "deconstructing cravings". Perhaps we are yearning to just experience the joy of a childhood memory again, or maybe we just want to be transported back to a favorite vacation where all the food was simply amazing: the soups of Peru, the guacamole of Costa Rica, the Mojito's of Cuba...you get the idea.

Even though the food we eat has the power to transport us back in time, we have to make real-time choices. Our bodies might not be able to tolerate certain foods anymore. Face it, food isn't what it used to be. All those chemicals, GMOs, and processed foods wreak havoc on our digestive systems. Eating healthy is more challenging than ever before. The search for organic fruits, vegetables, and meat and fish that are treated humanely and raised without antibiotics is crucial to our health.

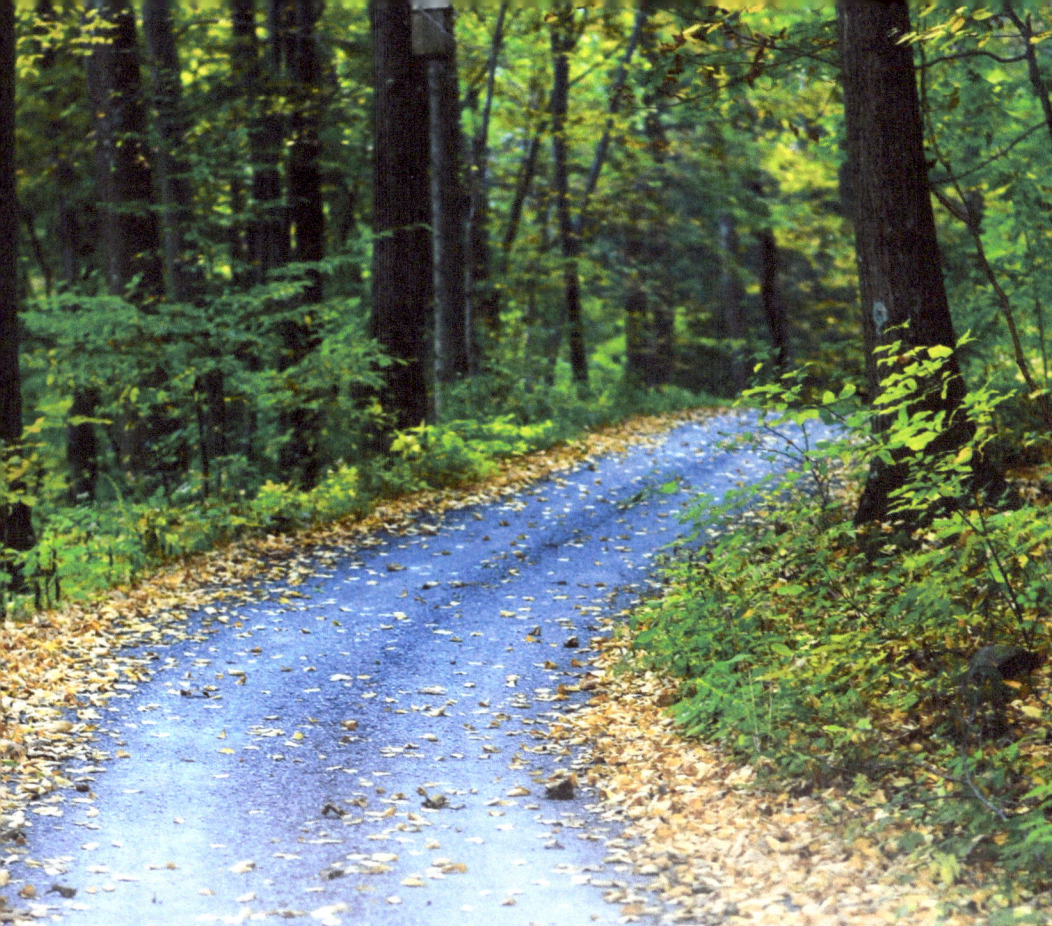

I read somewhere that every time you take a bite, you are either breaking down or building up your body. Food is medicine, but today's food can also be a poison. It's more important than ever to be conscious of our choices. If you are reading this book, then something inside you is already searching for a better way of eating and a healthier lifestyle.

Every choice we make and every bite we take can affect how our body will function. The exciting new research in the field of epigenetics, in a nutshell, simply says, "The diet and lifestyle we choose has a direct impact on how our genes express themselves." For instance, just because so many people in my family have diabetes doesn't mean I have to be doomed to get it. Yes, if I eat like them I will have a greater chance of heading in that direction. But, if I change my lifestyle and eating habits, the chances are significantly less. If you are worried about going down the same road as some of your family members, then you need to choose another road.

Zucchini Bread

It counts as a veggie, right?

During the peak of zucchini season, there's no end to what you can make with them. Everything from grilled zucchini, zucchini cheesy bread, zucchini soup, to one of my family's favorites, zucchini bread. Not every recipe in this book is necessarily super healthy (because of the sugar content), but what's not to love about homemade zucchini bread. I switch it up and alternate between the regular bread and a "death by chocolate" version. There are also times when there are so many zucchinis ready at one time that I take advantage of the surplus and freeze some for out-of-season baking. All you have to do is grate fresh zucchini and freeze it in two cup amounts. When you want to make one of these bread recipes, just defrost the zucchini and use it in the recipe. It's that easy; and there's nothing better in the dead of winter than a warm slice of this bread with a cup of hot tea.

Regular Version:

2 cups sugar
1 cup vegetable oil
3 eggs
2 cups grated zucchini
3 1/2 cups flour
1/2 tsp. vanilla; 1/2 tsp. salt
2 tsp. baking soda
1/2 tsp. nutmeg; 1/2 tsp. cinnamon
2 cups raisins; 1 cup chopped nuts

Begin by mixing oil and sugar together with an electric mixer. Add eggs, zucchini, flour, and spices. Mix well. Add raisins and nuts.

Pour equally into two greased bread pans.

Bake at 350 degrees for about 55 minutes. Makes 2 loaves.

Chocolate Version:

1 1/4 cup flour; 1/2 c. cocoa powder
1 tsp. baking soda
1 tsp. cinnamon; 1/4 tsp. salt
1 cup sugar; 1 egg plus 1 egg yolk
1/2 c. melted butter; 1 tsp. vanilla extract
2 cups grated zucchini
2/3 cup chocolate chips (optional)

Whisk together flour, cocoa powder, baking soda, cinnamon, and salt.

In another bowl, stir together sugar and eggs. Add melted butter and vanilla extract and mix until smooth. Add zucchini and mix again. Add flour mixture and beat until smooth. Fold in chocolate chips.

Transfer to a baking pan that has been greased and dusted with a little cocoa powder. Bake at 350 degrees for 45-50 minutes. Makes 1 loaf.

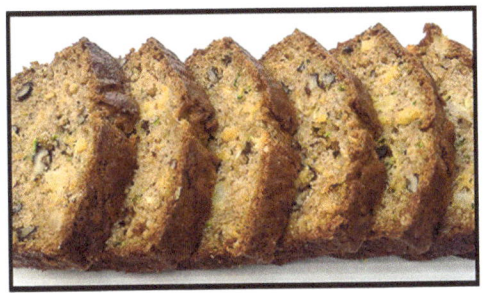
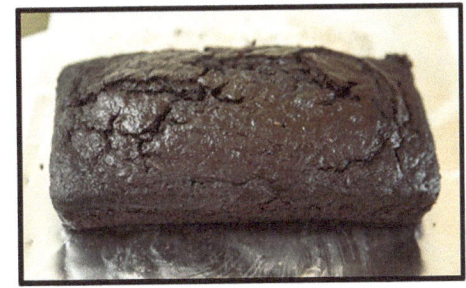

Food for Thought!

Zucchini is high in the heart-healthy mineral potassium. One cup of cooked zucchini gives you more than 15 percent of your daily value. Zucchini includes a lot of fiber called pectin, which is a type of beneficial polysaccharide that is linked to improved cardiovascular health and the ability to lower cholesterol naturally. Zucchini offers a good dose of phytonutrients like vitamin C, manganese, beta carotene, lutein and zeaxanthin that protect eye health. Zucchini and other types of summer squash are often recommended for digestive issues and diverticulitis since they're hydrating and provide essential electrolytes and nutrients.

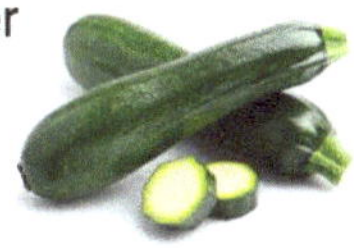

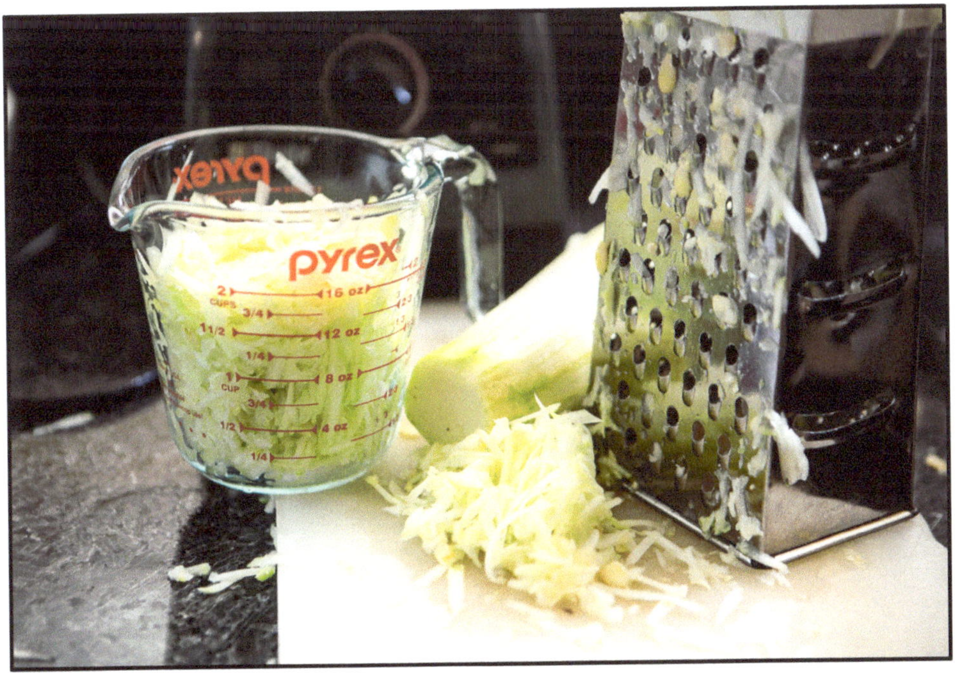

Just Breathe

Sometimes all it takes is the smell of something sweet and wonderful to fill our hearts with joy.

A breath in, a breath out. We do it every second of our lives without a second thought. From the moment we took our first breath as a newborn to our dying breath as we leave this world, it's our constant companion. When was the last time you took a deep breath? One that started in your toes, expanded your belly, filled your chest, and touched the tippity top of your head.

When we take a deep purposeful breath, the diaphragm massages the stomach, small intestine, liver and pancreas. The upper movement of the diaphragm also massages the heart. When we inhale, our diaphragm descends and our belly expands. When this happens, we massage vital organs and improve circulation in them. Mindful breathing releases stress that gets built up in the body. Stress sends a message to our body to hold off on functions that are not essential, such as digestion, until our body is safe to rest and repair. This means that digestion often takes a back seat, leaving us more vulnerable to inflammation and disease.

In today's high paced world, our adrenals need a break. We can activate our parasympathetic nervous system through the simple act of deep breathing exercises.

Think about how breathing can enhance our cooking experience, too. A deep breath of a freshly cut sprig of rosemary on a cutting board, the aroma of soup simmering on the cook top, the smell of cinnamon and sweet apples as a pie bakes in the oven, all wake up our senses.

When was the last time you just closed your eyes, took a deep breath, and gave thanks for the richness of the food we are blessed with?

The Perfect Recipe

Some things you just can't measure

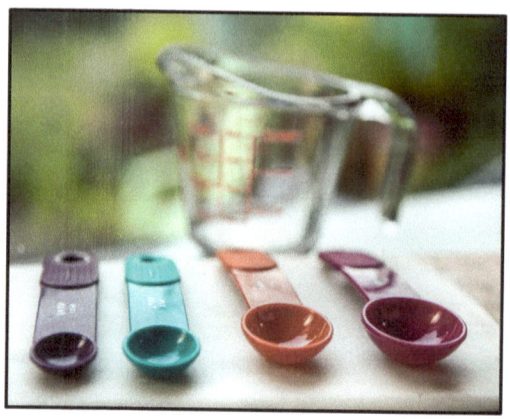

My mother drove me absolutely crazy! That statement may have applied to many situations, but what I'm referring to is her ability to bake without a recipe. My mom wasn't the best cook in the world. She knew two stove settings: off and high. The only real spices I knew growing up were salt and pepper. When it was time for dinner, I drove her nuts; I wouldn't eat hardly anything. However, when it came to either baked goods or Polish foods, she was in her element. Kiffles, pierogies, apple pie, to name just a few, were mouthwatering. I can't be the only one who can tell a story like this.

It was when I was in my early twenties that I first became interested in duplicating some of her recipes and trying them on my own. I'd ask her for the recipe, and this is where the madness began. She'd pull a glass out of the cupboard. There would be some random scratch half way up the glass. She'd hold it up and proudly say, "Use this glass and fill sugar up to the scratch." What! It drove me crazy. I'd say, "Well how much is that?" I did the only thing I could possibly do. I poured the sugar into said glass, then poured that amount into a real measuring cup. Aah! One half cup. Now we were getting somewhere. This didn't happen just one time. Over and over again, it was using a scratch in a glass for this, or a handful of that.

Mom's apple pie was one of those wonders. There literally was no written-down recipe. Not a measuring spoon in sight. It was just a handful of this, and a sprinkling of that. After watching her bake these pies over the years, I'm proud to say that I can duplicate that recipe perfectly without a measuring spoon in sight. Now it's my handful of this or that that lovingly gets sprinkled into the mix.

What I discovered after all these years is that my mom's ability to intuitively know what to add to a dish and how much to add was really something very empowering. I've embraced that now. I'm so proud when I cook with fearless abandonment. I always encourage my cooking classes to be a bit daring. Listen to your gut and be guided by your nose. What's the worst that could happen? You won't like what you cooked, and then you won't make it that way again. No big deal.

With that said, I'm going to share with you the best apple pie recipe ever!

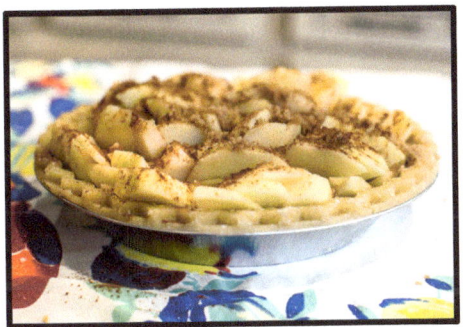

Mom's Apple Pie

Take one handful of flour and sprinkle it on the bottom of a pie crust. I actually use a store-bought pie crust. There is no need to defrost it before making the pie. Add one handful of sugar to the flour and then sprinkle in a generous amount of cinnamon to the sugar/flour combination.

Take your finger and swirl the flour, sugar, and cinnamon together so the entire bottom of the crust is covered. Mom always used her finger and never a spatula.

Peel apples (any type of baking apple is fine; McIntosh or Jonathan). Place apple slices all around the pie crust until it is entirely filled. About 5-6 apples per pie.

Pour 1/4 cup of water over the apples. This is the only thing I actually measure! Add one handful of sugar over the apples and then add one handful of brown sugar over that. Sprinkle pie with a generous amount of cinnamon. Add 4-5 small thin pats of butter around the pie.

Bake at 375 degrees for about 45-50 minutes or until apples are soft when poked with a fork. Time will vary depending on thickness of apple slices and type of apple.

Time to go Nuts

Soaking nuts offers health benefits

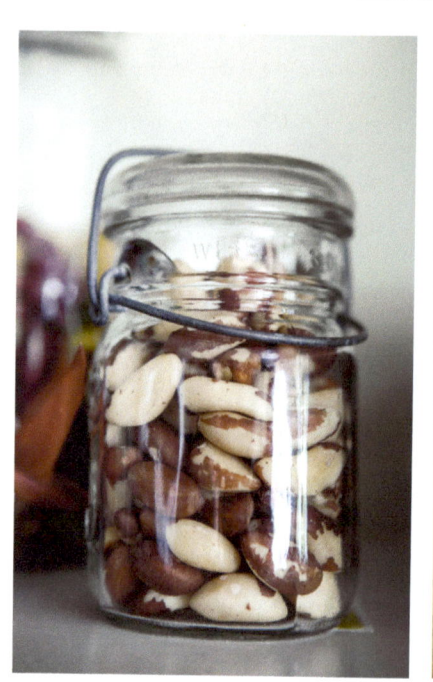
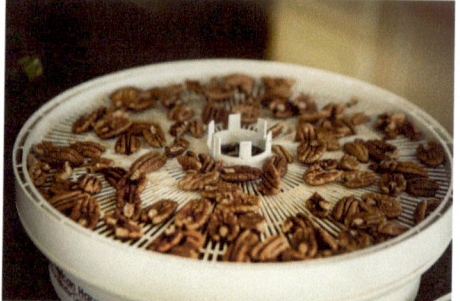
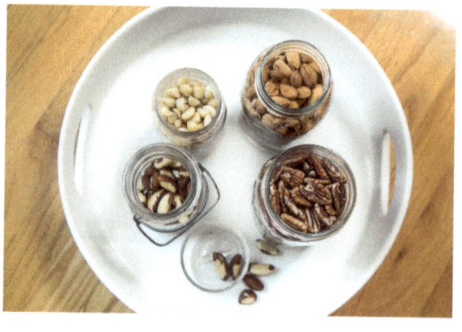

When it comes to a quick and healthy snack, it's hard to beat a handful of nuts. One of the best things about nuts is their high content of healthy fats. Nuts are a wonderful source of omega-3 fatty acids, more specifically, alpha-linoleic acid. This type of fatty acid has certain anti-inflammatory properties that have been shown to reduce the chances of colon, prostate, and breast cancer. Another plus is that the high level of dietary fiber in nuts promotes good bowel movements and digestion, which reduces the chances of certain types of gastrointestinal cancers. Almonds help balance cholesterol and improve insulin sensitivity. Macadamia nuts boost heart health and reduce inflammation. Pecans boost antioxidant levels, and Walnuts provide omega-3 and balance cholesterol and blood pressure. All of these benefits are great, but you have to be careful to choose raw organic nuts and prepare them properly.

If there's one negative about nuts, it's that they contain something called phytic acid. Phytic acid is also found in grains and legumes. Just like you should soak grains and legumes, soaking nuts is essential for proper digestion. When eating nuts that haven't been soaked, the phytic acid binds to minerals in your intestinal tract and cannot be absorbed in the intestines properly. By soaking nuts in salted water for 12 to 24 hours, you break down the phytic acid so it can be absorbed properly. Soaking also helps reduce the number of lectins that are present in nuts. Lectins can also wreak havoc on your digestive system.

Here's what to do:

1. Pour raw, unsalted, organic nuts/seeds into a large glass bowl.

2. Cover with filtered water so that nuts are submerged and covered with at least an extra inch of water. (they will puff up)

3. Add 1-2 tablespoons unrefined salt.

4. Let nuts soak covered on the kitchen counter for about 7 hours, or overnight.

5. Rinse nuts to remove salt residue and spread out in single layer on a rack to dehydrate.

6. Dry at a low temperature (generally no higher than 150 degrees) in dehydrator or oven for 12-24 hours or until nuts are slightly crispy. Make sure the nuts are really dry or they will get moldy.

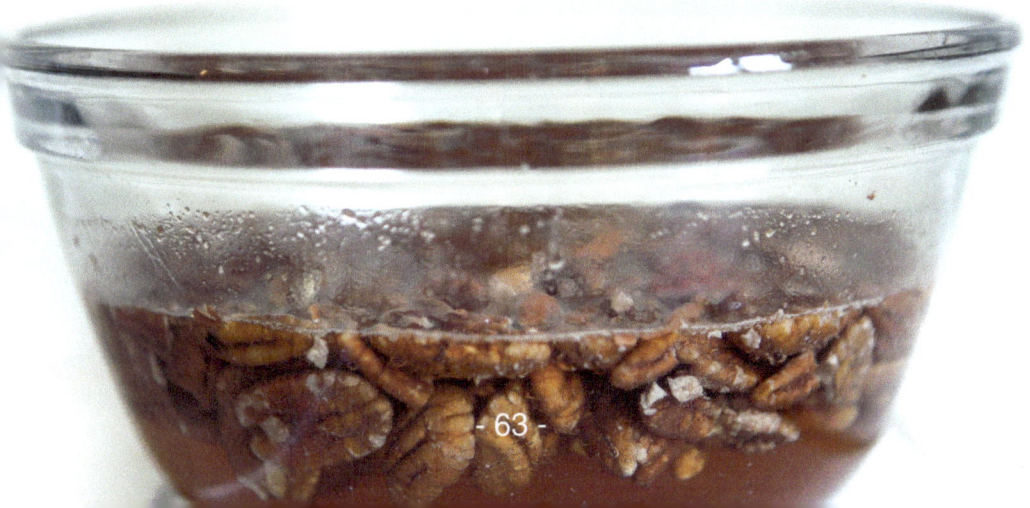

Ritual vs. Habit

Peeling Back the Layers

Table for One

Preserve Family Traditions

Honor a Simple Choice

At the End of the Day

Winter

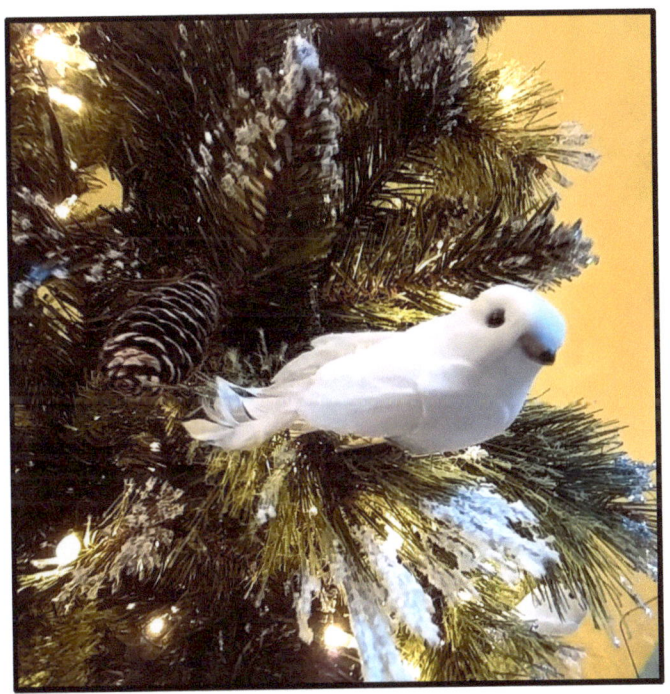

Cherish the gifts that life gives us

In the Still of Winter

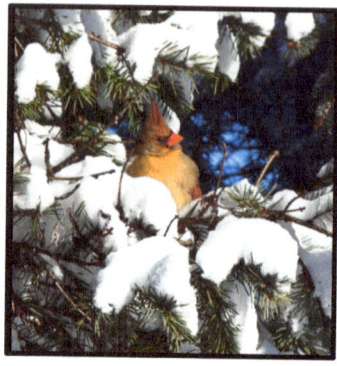

Snow falling on the pines, benches covered in fluffy pillows of white, the sound of quiet blankets the landscape. It's beautiful.... if you like snow. Winters in the Northeast have a way of testing the fortitude of the strongest of spirits. People either love it or hate it. It's pretty black and white, literally. For people like me who really struggle with winter, learning to make the best of the season is a real challenge. I must admit, though, that I do love a freshly fallen snow, as long as I don't have to drive in it, and everyone I care about is safe at home. In all seriousness, winter is just what the body needs after a busy summer and fall. Just like flowers go into hibernation to prepare for another season, and animals hunker down, our bodies need time to rest and recuperate. Learning to honor that need isn't always easy. Everyone complains about how it gets dark so early, but that darkness offers us a chance to settle in early, put on our jammies, make a hot cup of tea and curl up with a good book or movie.

Just as our activities change in the winter, so should our eating habits. The need to eat for the seasons is vitally important. Our bodies instinctively crave comfort food in winter. Foods like root vegetables that have been growing underground all summer soaking up all that awesome earth energy help us stay grounded during these long cold months. Steaming hot soups and hearty chili warm our bodies from the inside out, like a warm and fuzzy hug. A higher fat diet during this time provides insulation and nutrients that we need to repair, rebuild, and rejuvenate before spring comes.

Winter is also the perfect time for house projects that took a back seat during the summer. Clean out a closet, reorganize that junk drawer, take on that paint project that's been on the back burner. Or hey, just go out and build a snowman!

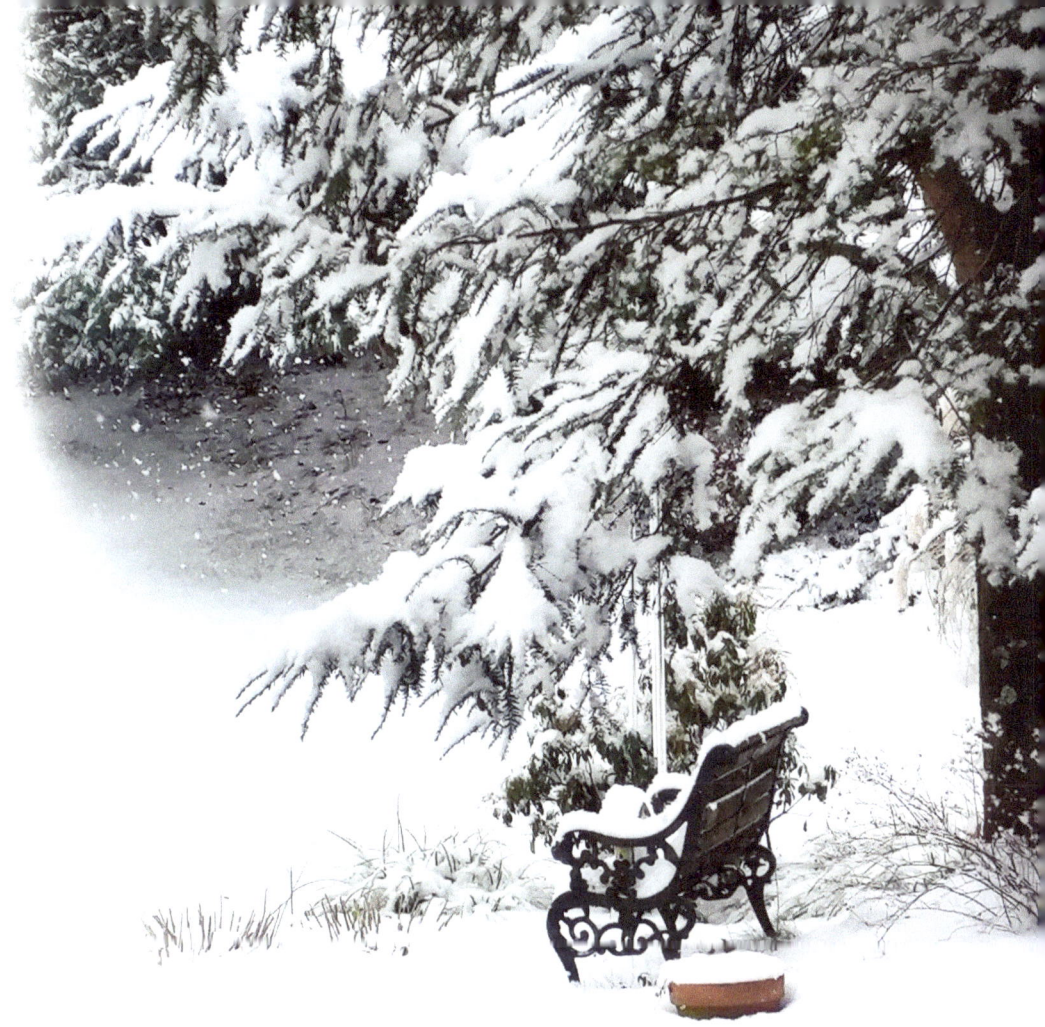

Warm and delicious apple treat

A super easy dessert that's also healthy is warmed spiced apples. If it were any other season, just grabbing a crispy cold apple would sound inviting. But in winter, not so much. This treat is so simple. Just take an apple or two and slice it into thin pieces. Layer the slices in a glass baking dish. Sprinkle cinnamon and nutmeg over the apple slices. Add a handful of raisins and nuts for over-the-top goodness. Dot with a pat of butter and add just enough water so the apples won't stick to the dish. Bake at 350 degrees until apples are soft, about 20 minutes. I often make this in a small dish just for me. It's so easy and so good!

Good morning world . . .

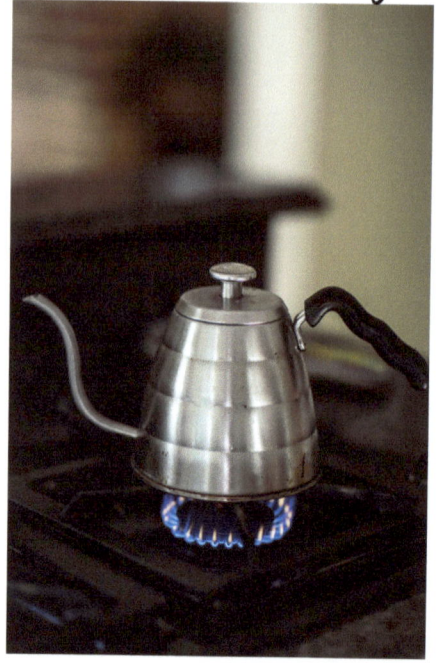
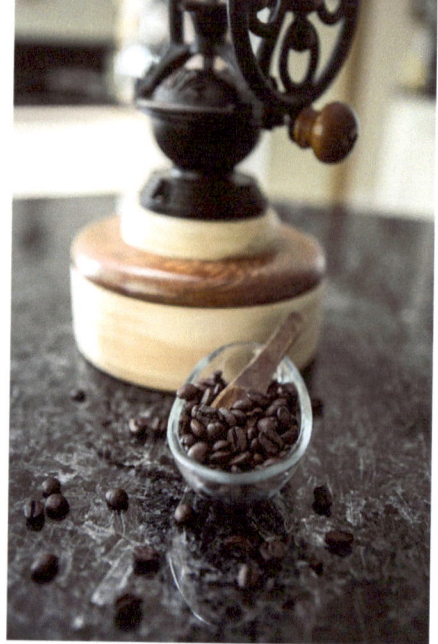
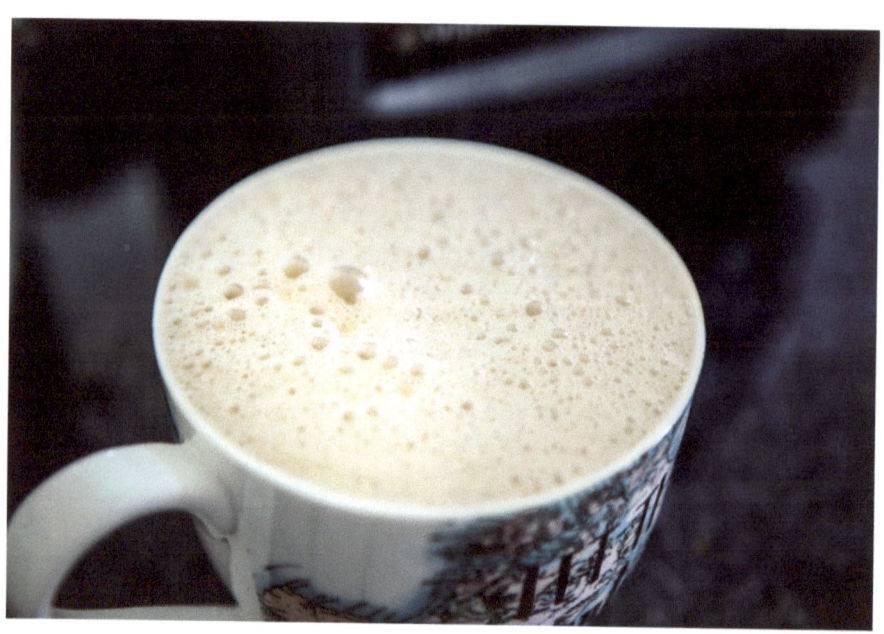

Ritual vs. Habit

Ritual vs. habit..... so, what's the real difference? To me a habit is something we do mindlessly without thinking about it too much. It's like being on auto pilot. It slips by without a true beginning, middle, and ending. There's nothing really special about a habit; we take it for granted and pay little attention to it. Take making your morning coffee for instance. You wander sleepily into the kitchen. Still groggy from a restless night's sleep, you flip on the coffee machine and stare into space until the first sip hits your lips. It's a habit which many of us can relate to. We do it every day. Day after day. Without a second thought.

What if we were open to a new way of thinking about that morning coffee? What if...... we could take that "habit" and turn it into a ritual. We could turn it into something that was purposeful, meaningful, and deliberate. It would have a beginning, a middle, and a beautiful end result. It would be the only thing we focused on at that moment. The thought of multi-tasking would be simply out of the question.

What if suddenly all the sounds and aromas of this ritual spoke to us, saying, "It's time to wake up, time to start our day, time to give gratitude for having another day, and time to live this day with purpose." How cool would that experience be! The day would be off to such an awesome start. Don't worry tea drinkers, all this applies to you, too.

From the first click of the gas burner igniting, to the steam rising over the coffee grinds, to the first delicious sip that hits our lips, this simple act of making coffee becomes, in a way, a prayer in motion. Now this ordinary habit turns into a ritual that is a deliberate act of self-care and nourishment.

White Chicken Chili

This delicious chicken chili was the hit of my winter chili cooking class. Absolutely everyone raved about it. It's creamy, savory, and hearty; just what your body needs in the dead of winter to keep you warm from the inside out. You can control the amount of heat by cutting down or adding more cayenne pepper and green chilies. The sour cream and heavy cream combination make this dish so silky smooth and rich. This recipe is a great alternative to the traditional red chili we grew up with as a kid.

You're gonna need:

1 medium onion, chopped
1 yellow and 1 red pepper, seeded and chopped
4 cloves garlic, minced
1 tbsp. olive oil
1 or 2 (4oz.) cans chopped green chilies (depends on spice level preference)
1 lb. boneless organic chicken breasts cut into bite size pieces
2 (14 oz.) cans great northern beans, drained and rinsed
14 oz. chicken broth
1 tsp. salt
1 tsp. ground cumin
1 tsp. oregano
1/2 tsp. pepper
1/4 tsp. cayenne pepper
8 oz. sour cream
1/2 cup whipping or heavy cream

Here's what to do:

Sauté the onion, garlic, and peppers in butter, ghee, or olive oil (your choice) until tender. Add the diced chilies and sauté a few minutes longer. Add the diced chicken pieces and cook until chicken is fully cooked.

Combine chicken, onions, garlic, and peppers together with the chicken broth and then add all the spices and the 2 cans of beans.

Simmer for 20 to 30 minutes. Remove from heat and add the sour cream and heavy cream. Serve immediately and feel all warm inside.

In the isolation of winter, nature rests. Time seems to stand still, frozen in a moment of silent introspection. So, it is with us, too. Resist the urge to "do something". Be still and listen to your inner voice. Therein lies the beauty of the soul.

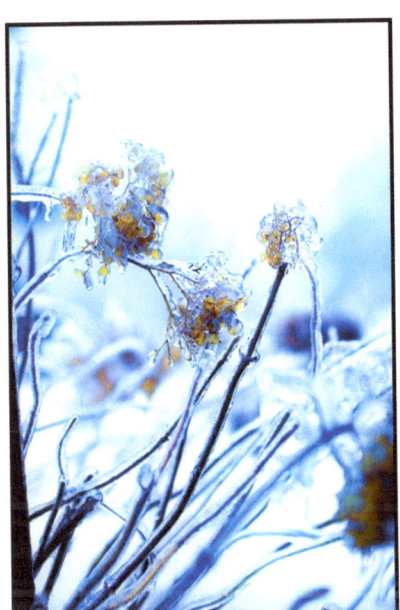
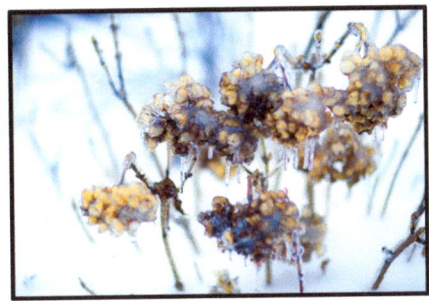
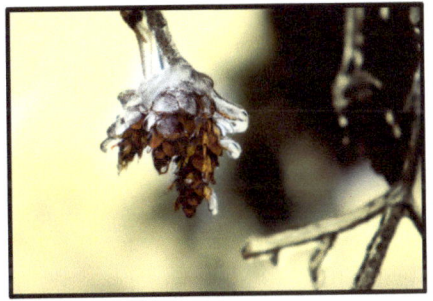
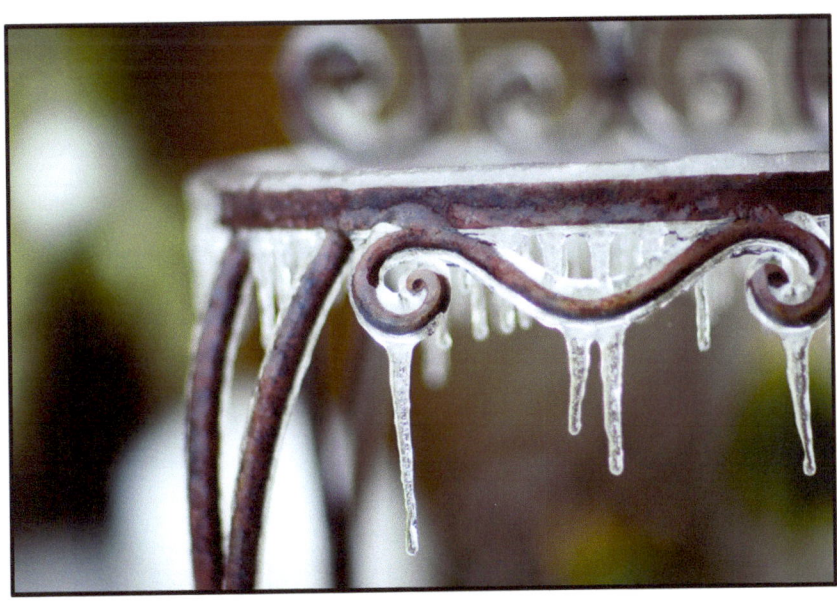

Peeling Back the Layers

Discovering the path to healthy eating

Taking responsibility for our health should be our number one priority. It's a commitment to honoring ourselves with every mouthful we consume and every action we take. It isn't easy and sometimes not even fun. For some of us, we live in total denial of how our decisions impact us. How many times have I heard, "Ya gotta die of something!" That's true, but why sabotage our chances of simply dying of old age. Why stack the odds against us?

It's so easy to eat wrong. America has made it super convenient. Just pick up a pizza here, grab a sandwich there, drop a dollar in a vending machine for a quick pick me up; do I need to go on? Usually it takes some kind of wake-up call to change eating habits. It could be something a relative or close friend is going through that makes us take a look at ourselves, or it could be a visit to a doctor for an annual exam and not hearing the kind of results that we hoped. For me, it was a combination of things: the birth of my grandson and the desire to be around for his wedding, the in-your-face reality of watching my much older brothers and sisters deal with the problems of aging, and the genetic disposition of my parents. We all have our reasons that finally push us to take the first step towards making better decisions.

It starts small. I use the visual of an onion when I think about the process of making better eating choices. When that first layer of the onion gets peeled off, it's the first step to getting to its core. An example might be this: You decide to give up soda or soft drinks. You feel good about making that decision. It's hard, but you are willing to do it. So instead you choose to drink iced tea. This feels good for a while; after all, it's much better than all that sugar in soda. But then something else starts to happen. You are willing to peel away another layer on that onion. All of a sudden you begin to think that maybe that sweetened ice tea isn't the best thing to drink either. Eventually you make the decision to drink unsweetened ice tea, and after that plain water, and finally you start adding a lemon to the water to affect the alkalinity of your body. You are on the road to making great decisions.

But it doesn't stop there. Once you start giving up the obvious list of junk food items that just about everyone knows isn't really good for you, you turn your focus to fresh fruits and vegetables. That choice is so much better than anything that comes in a box. For a long time, making that shift feels incredibly empowering. Then it starts again. Off comes another layer of that onion. This time you take a look at exactly which fruits and vegetables are right for you. Not for everyone else, but just you. What if you love tomatoes but they cause inflammation in your joints. What if carrots are full of so much nutrition but they wreak havoc on your sugar levels. Now those wonderful fresh vegetables are put on the do-not-eat list. Going down the rabbit hole to health is a journey. It's a never-ending process of decision making and soul searching for our individual recipe for vibrant health. We have to follow our gut; we have the answers inside. We just have to love ourselves enough to fight for what is right for us.

Every layer we uncover is taking us to the core of who we really are.

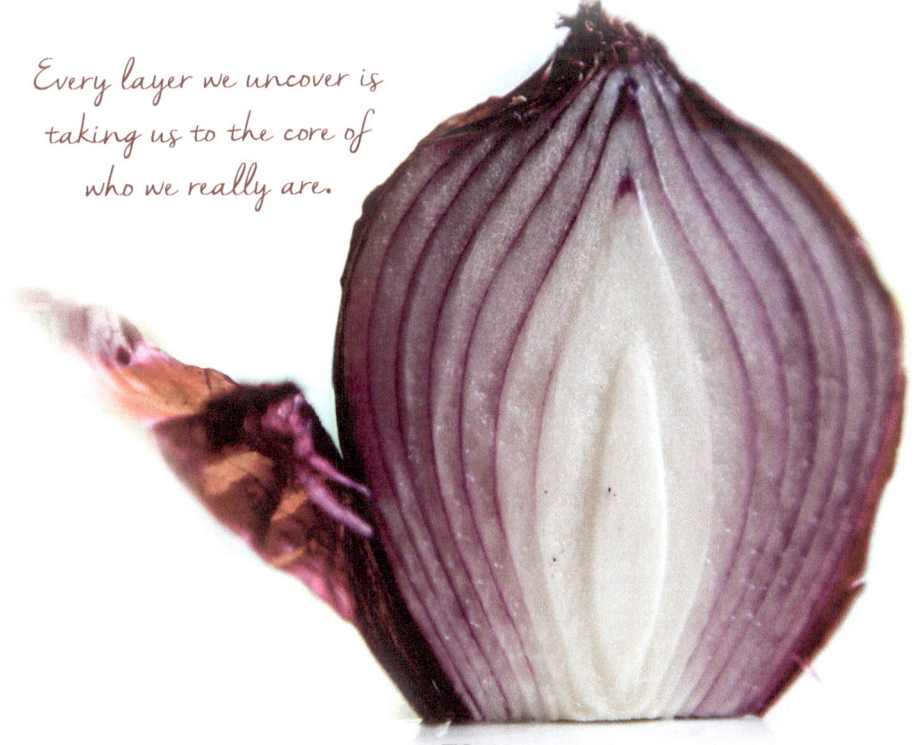

Sweet Potato Bisque

This is one of my absolute favorite soups. It's creamy, with a blend of sweet and savory. Rosemary and garlic marry into an absolutely amazing taste. Inspired by a recipe from the book "If the Buddha Came to Dinner", it's a hit any time of year. I love to go out to the garden to pick the rosemary right from the garden and the kale that is added at the very end comes right off the tower garden on the back deck. It's totally vegan, so that's a plus.

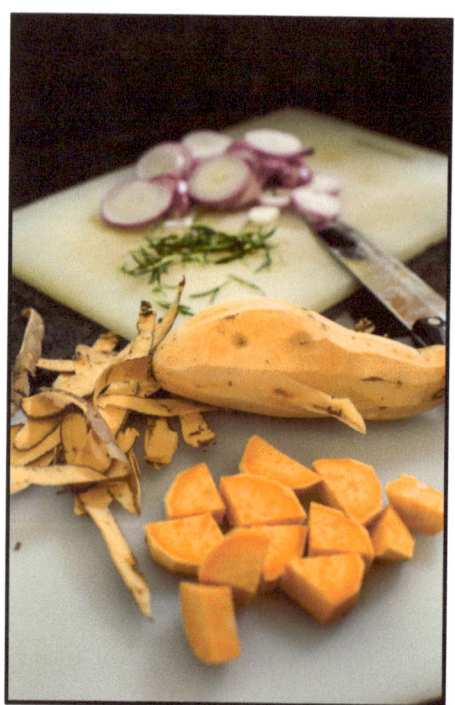

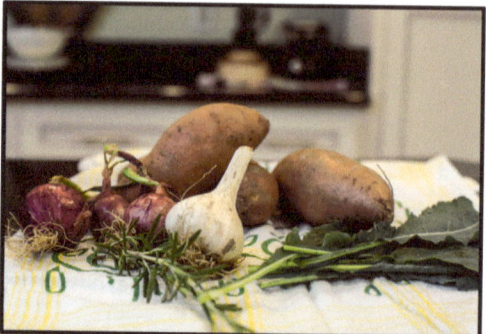

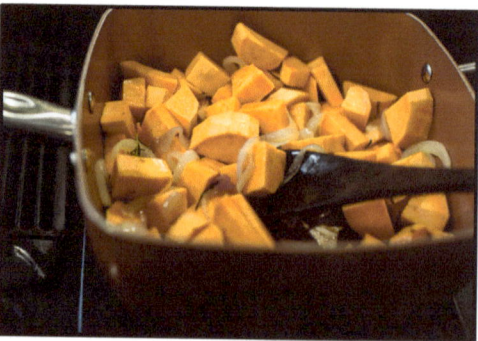

Food for Thought!

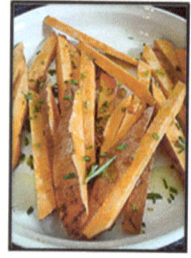

Sweet potatoes help stabilize blood sugar, boost brain function, enhance immunity, promote vision health and are high in antioxidants. Sweet potatoes are jam-packed with vitamin A, which supports our immunity.

For sweet potato fries, simply slice unpeeled sweet potatoes, sprinkle with fresh rosemary, and drizzle with olive oil. Bake at 400 degrees for about 25-30 minutes, or use an air fryer to make them extra crispy. YUM!

You're gonna need:

1 entire head of garlic

4 small leeks or shallots (both work great)

2 sprigs of rosemary

4 cups of peeled and diced sweet potatoes

4 cups vegetable stock

salt and pepper to taste

fresh kale, chopped into tiny pieces

Here's what to do:

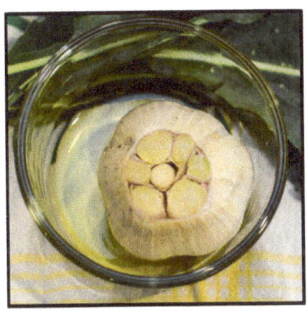

HOW TO PREP THE GARLIC: Trim the top off the head of garlic. Place the entire head in a small glass baking dish. Drizzle olive oil over the garlic. Cover and bake at 300 degrees for about 30 minutes. Remove from oven and let cool just enough so you can handle it. Remove the garlic cloves from the casings and chop the cloves into tiny bits.

While the garlic is baking, peel the sweet potatoes and cut into small pieces. Peel and chop the shallots or leeks. Make sure the leeks are really clean. Strip the rosemary from its stalk and chop into tiny bits.

Pour about two tablespoons of olive oil into your soup pot. Sauté shallots (or leeks) along with the rosemary until tender. Add the diced sweet potatoes. This is the time for the shallots, rosemary and sweet potatoes to get to know each other. The olive oil, shallots and rosemary get to coat the sweet potatoes and become friends. Stir occasionally. After about 5 minutes, add the vegetable stock.

Cover, and let the soup cook at a gentle rolling boil for about 25 minutes, or until sweet potatoes are soft. Using an immersion blender, puree soup until silky smooth. Salt and pepper to taste. Add the chopped kale immediately before serving. It will wilt quickly.

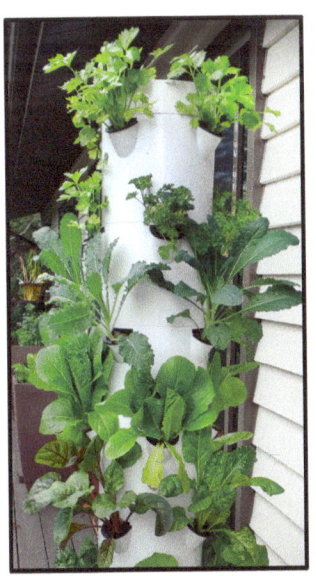

Vegetables are so easy to grow with this tower garden. Veggies grow with air and water. No soil!

If you think the soup is too thick, just add more stock.

Table for One
You're worth making dinner for!

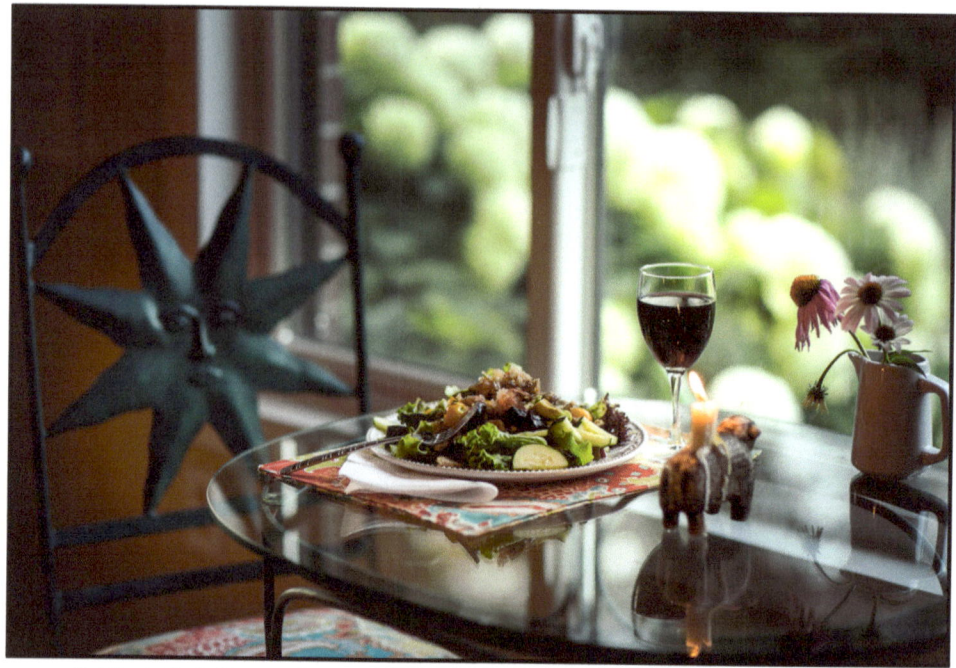

Set the table, light a candle, pour a glass of wine, open the window, and listen to the birds.

If I had a dollar for every time I heard, "Oh, I don't cook. It's only me." I'd be able to buy enough organic produce to last a lifetime! I get it. Nine out of ten meals that I cook are just for myself, and there's plenty of times that I don't feel like going through the effort just for me. I came to realize, however, that I'm worth it. I'm worth having amazing food to eat. I deserve food that nourishes my body so that I can provide for those I love. There are so many ways to rationalize the argument that, yes, if you are preparing meals for yourself, you shouldn't have to go through all that effort. But what if you were open to a new possibility? The possibility that creating meals for yourself doesn't have to be hard; the possibility that those meals could actually be equally as enjoyable as sharing a meal with friends or family, and the possibility that those meals might not take as much time and effort as you think. With just a few tricks, these possibilities can become a reality.

So what are the tricks that make meal prep for yourself easier? First of all, cook one meal that could easily feed four people. What? Yes! Cook like you are feeding a family. Place a huge batch of veggies on a baking sheet, drizzle with olive oil and seasonings and bake until the veggies are perfect. It's not rocket science. What you don't eat at your first meal, becomes delicious leftovers for quick lunches or snacks. These veggies could also serve as a great base for the beginning of another quick meal. Think of them as volunteers for a new dish. Be fearless about combining these leftovers with just one new item; the combinations are endless. This is one reason I love soup so much. You go through the effort once, but can enjoy that soup for multiple meals. The more premade meals that are in your refrigerator, the greater the chance of eating healthy will be. There's a standing joke between a friend and me about rotisserie chicken that you can buy at the grocery store. First it becomes a main meal, the next day part of it turns up in a salad, by the third day any leftovers readily jump into a big pot of chicken soup. The best part is that I didn't even have to cook the chicken in the first place to reap all the benefits. These are just a few samples of what you can do. Just remember, you are worth it!

Preserve Family Traditions

The tradition of making Christmas cookies runs deep in my family. I fondly remember making them with my mother. We would always cut them out in the exact same order. We cut out all the playing card shapes first: aces, hearts, diamonds, spades. Next would be Santas, leaves, and bells. It was unthinkable to start in any other order! After my mother passed, my sister and I carried on the tradition. Oh, and did I mention we always had to bake with Christmas carols by Bing Crosby playing in the background? Any other music was just sacrilegious.

Although my sister and I still bake together, the family tradition took an unexpected turn. My son decided to continue the tradition with his wife and two of their buddies. My son is a huge collector of all things comic, horror, and sports related memorabilia; and this obsession/fascination to this genre was evident at his cookie making night. Now Bing Crosby is replaced with the movie Silent Night, Deadly Night playing in the background. And those cute Santa cutouts of my mother's era turned into Freddie Krueger cutouts. Some people may be offended by this and think it's disturbing, but the thing is, I'm ok with it. I actually embrace it because he's creating his own tradition. My grandson will think this is perfectly normal and cool, and it is. It is because the act of engaging in and creating family traditions feeds our soul. I don't even like these cookies, but I love making them because of all the sweet memories it brings back. Over and over again, I stress that our total health depends not only on the actual food we eat, but soooooo many other factors. Family traditions are an integral part of our relationship area of our lives.

The more we nurture our relationships, the stronger the support of our total health becomes. Nurturing relationships isn't restricted to boyfriends, girlfriends, or spouses. Relationships extend to our friends, coworkers, neighbors, social groups, and yes, our families. Take time to develop new relationships and make existing ones stronger, and see how much better you feel. And when you're feeling better, you'll be able to enjoy all those traditions to the fullest no matter how wacky they are.

MORE THAN A CUTOUT COOKIE

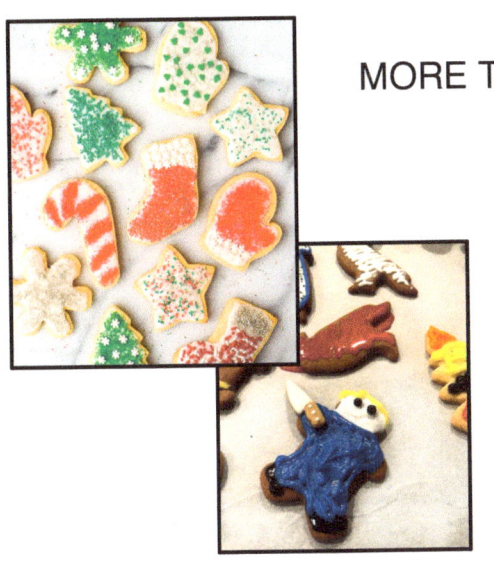

You're gonna need:

Use an electric mixer to combine:

1 1/2 c. sugar

1 c. softened butter

3 eggs

1/2 tsp. salt

1 tsp. baking soda

1 tsp. vanilla

After mixing the above ingredients, slowly add 4 1/2 c. flour a little bit at a time until it's all combined. At this point, you might have to knead it by hand to mix it all up. If the dough still sticks to your fingers, you just keep sprinkling more flour into the bowl until the dough comes off your fingers easily and isn't super sticky. I always end up adding more flour than what is called for.

Form the dough into small loaves and refrigerate at least overnight before baking cookies. The dough will roll out much easier if it is cold.

I use a large wooden cutting board to roll out the dough. Sprinkle a generous amount of sugar (yes, sugar) on the board and roll the dough out until it is nice and thin.

Using cookie cutters, create all your favorite shapes. Use cookie sprinkles to decorate the tops or get creative with icing. Bake at 350 degrees for 7 to 9 minutes. This recipe makes about two trays of cookies, so double or triple the recipe depending on how many cookies you want to make. Eat just a few, leave some for Santa, and give the rest away!

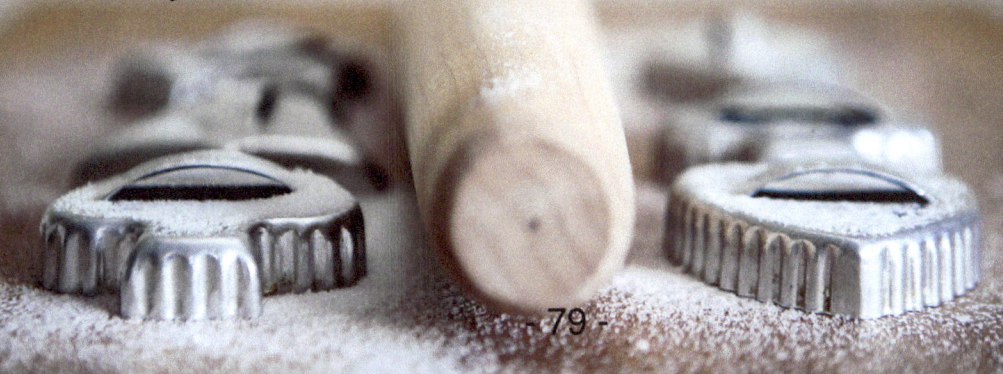

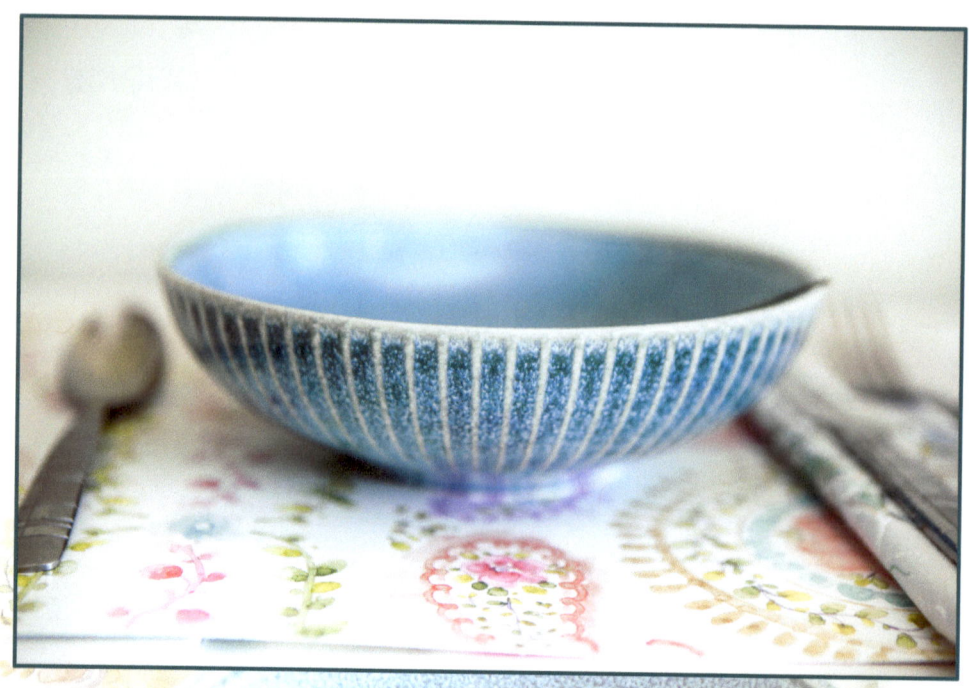

I grew up with dishes purchased week by week from the Acme grocery store. My mother would buy them a little at a time. Eventually, she bought a of set of them for me too. I bought lots of things in my life and splurged on more than a few luxury items, but I had a problem with spending money on dishes. God knows why!

Then one day I decided that I was worth a great set of new dishes. I ordered a whole set from my favorite potter, Royce Yoder. Everyone loved them. I did too. I still do. These dishes were not going to sit in the cupboard and come out on Sundays only. I love using them every day.

It wasn't until one of my dear friends suggested that, "Why not buy just one dish. Pick out one that speaks to you and use it whenever the mood strikes." And so, I did. It's fun mixing it up. Just like we change our jewelry with what we wear, using different plates, bowls, or cups makes what we are eating just a little more fun. What I discovered was that the ritual of selecting the bowl, plate, or cup became a journey in itself. What would that soup look good in? Which mug fits my mood today? From now on, every yard sale table and clearance rack are fair game.

Honor a simple choice

We all know that food fuels our bodies, but what we put that food in feeds much more than that. Choose your cup wisely my friends. With every sip that we take, those subliminal messages enter every cell of our body. Before we know it, things start happening if we just believe.

things happen for a reason.. just believe

"Selecting the bowl, plate, or cup became a journey in itself."

Cream of Broccoli Soup

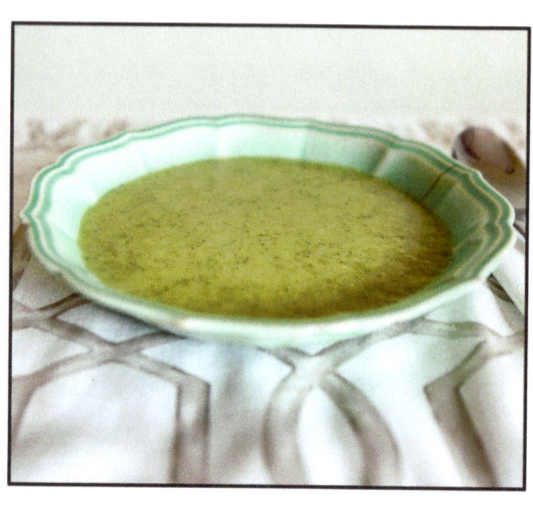

You're gonna need:

4 leeks, cleaned and diced thin

1 tbsp. avocado oil or ghee

3 c. chicken or vegetable stock

3 1/2 c. peeled and diced potatoes

4 c. broccoli florets

1/4 tsp. pepper

1 1/4 c. milk

1 c. grated Havarti cheese

salt to taste

Cream of broccoli soup is one of my very favorite soups. It's creamy and delicious; and with all that broccoli, it's packed with nutrients. Did you know that one cup of cooked broccoli has as much vitamin C as an orange? Broccoli, like many other cruciferous vegetables, contains abundant amounts of the carotenoid anti-oxidants lutein and zeaxanthin. These anti-oxidants help preserve eye function by slowing down age related macular degeneration, suppressing cataract development, and keeping healthy vision intact for years to come. It's also full of fiber and low in calories. It's a win-win combination.

One of the main reasons that I love soups so much is that it's such an easy meal when you are cooking for one person. You make it once and it lasts for several days. Having a healthy and hearty go-to meal really comes in handy when you either don't have time to cook or you just don't have the energy for it. Most soups also freeze well. You can take it out in the morning, and it's ready for lunch.

I've also experimented making this soup without adding milk and cheese when I was avoiding dairy for a while. It's still very good without the dairy; but in my opinion, cheese takes this soup over the top. You can also change it up by adding in some sautéed mushrooms. No matter what time of year it is, soup is easy and versatile. It's the perfect way to add goodness to your day.

Here's what to do:

Since leeks can be very sandy, it's super important to clean them thoroughly. Cut off all but about one inch of the green tops and discard the end roots. Make a long cut in the leeks about 1/2 of the way through the leek. This will allow you to open up the leek's layers and rinse the sand out. After you have all the dirt removed, slice the leeks into thin horizontal strips and set aside.

In a large soup pot, melt avocado oil or ghee (your choice). Add leeks and simmer until they are tender, about 10 minutes. Add a little stock if pot begins to dry out to prevent leeks from browning.

Add the potatoes, stock, and broccoli. Cover and cook over medium heat for about 25 minutes or until potatoes are soft. Using an immersion blender, puree soup until smooth. Add milk and grated cheese and stir until completely blended.

Simmer just long enough for cheese to melt and for the milk to get hot. If the soup is too thick, you can either add more milk or stock. This soup is also delicious without the milk and cheese as a vegan option.

Food for Thought!

A cup of cooked leeks contains 29% RDA of vitamin K. Vitamin K regulates clotting activities and transports calcium throughout the blood. Leeks also contain flavonoids and polyphenols, which assist in protecting both blood cells and vessels from oxidative damage. The primary flavonoid, kaempferol, is found in the lower leaf and bulb and is believed to protect the linings of blood vessels from damage. One cup of cooked leeks provides vitamins A, B6, C, E, and Omega-3 fatty acids, as well as manganese, copper, folate, and iron.

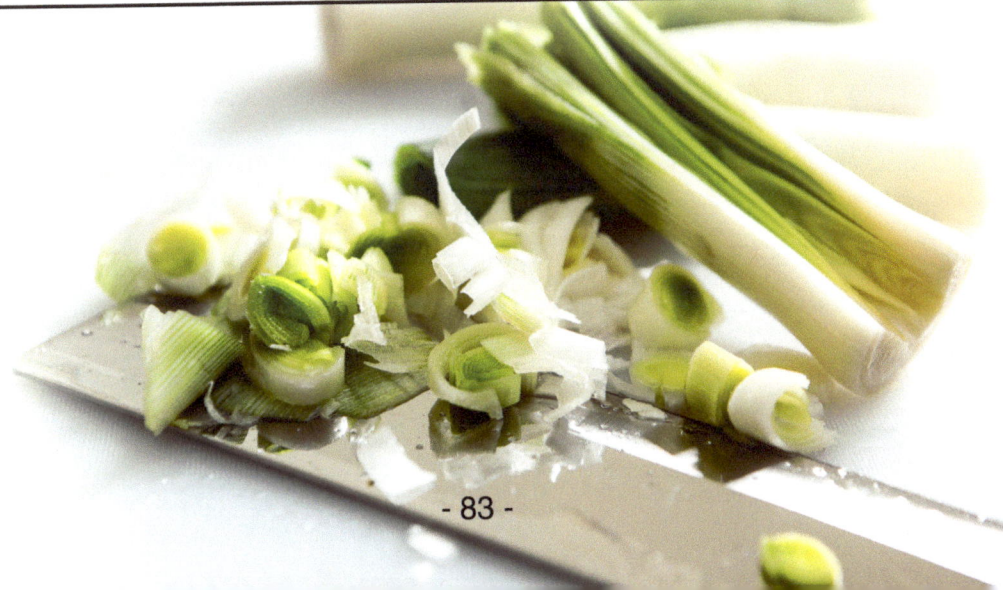

At the End of the Day

Taking stock of the life we live

At the end of the day, when we start the unwinding process of settling in for the night, the question remains, "What did we do for ourselves that truly added to our total health?" If we had a checklist, would our check marks land in the yes or no column? Review the day by asking, "Did I wake up in a state of gratitude?", if only to mumble, "Thank God I made it to another day." Even that simple thought points us in the right direction for the day. Was I aware of my daily habits, and with focus and intent, turn them into mindful rituals? Did I take time throughout the day to stop, breathe, and check in with what my body really needed? Did the foods I ate reflect my true desire to be healthy, or did I slip into old routines of careless eating?

Did I take time to play for a little bit? Whether it was with a child or a five-minute game of catch with a pet, play is important. Did I connect with others during the day? A chat with a neighbor, a Facebook message to a dear friend miles away, or a mid-day lunch with a co-worker are all valuable ways to bring a sense of relationship into our lives. Each and every one of these questions is important because they all stack the deck towards a healthier and happier lifestyle.

Did we chalk up today as a good day or a day we "cheated" with our eating habits? I always find it interesting that we use the word cheating when we fall off the proverbial food wagon. I wonder what would happen if we thought about all the good choices we made instead of the one or two bad ones. Whatever the answer is, we have to remember that we are only human. We're bound to make mistakes. We're bound to slip at times; and if we're lucky, we realize it. Hopefully, with some loving kindness towards ourselves, we pick ourselves up and take steps to make new choices that give us hope...choices that lead us to a longer and healthier life. And at the end of the day, when our tired bodies hit the pillow, will our last thought be, "Thank God for the gift of this day, and let nothing disturb the silence of this night."

Let nothing disturb

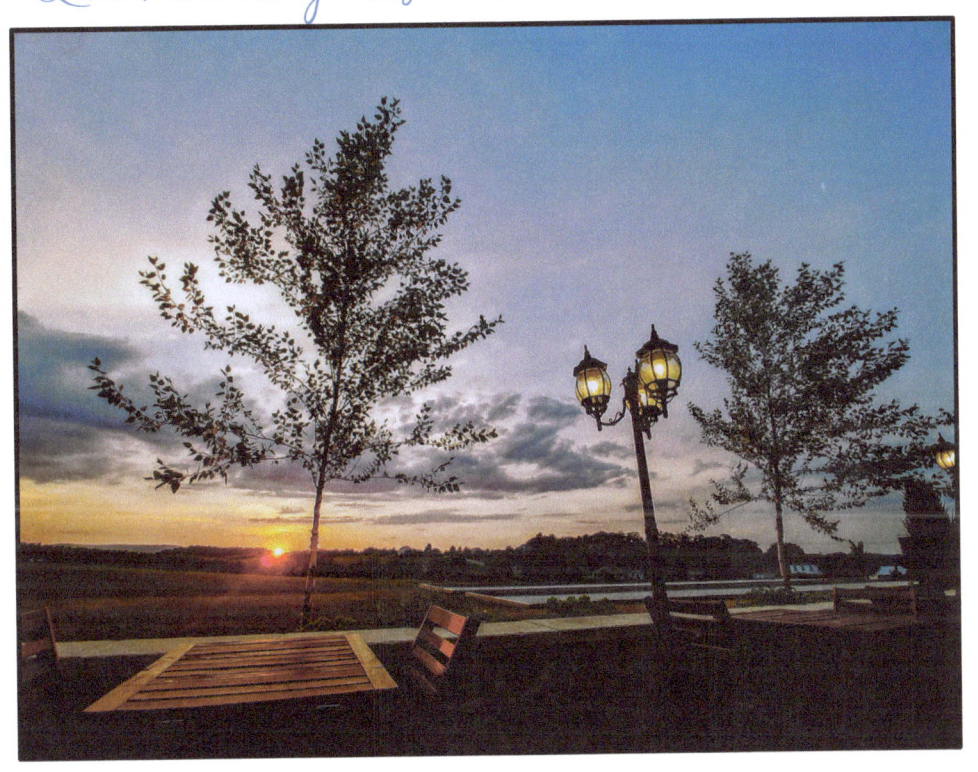

the silence of this night

Souper Sundays

How to Order an Apron

A Heartfelt Thank You

Favorite Gems to Shop

About IIN

In Addition

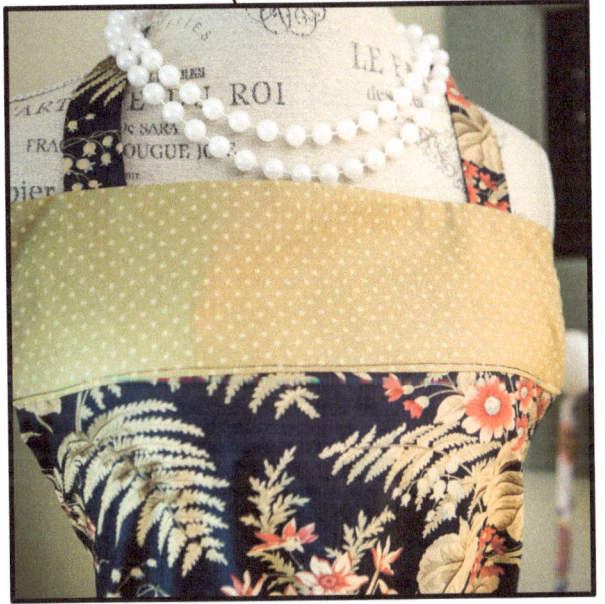

Good things you need to know

SOUPER SUNDAYS

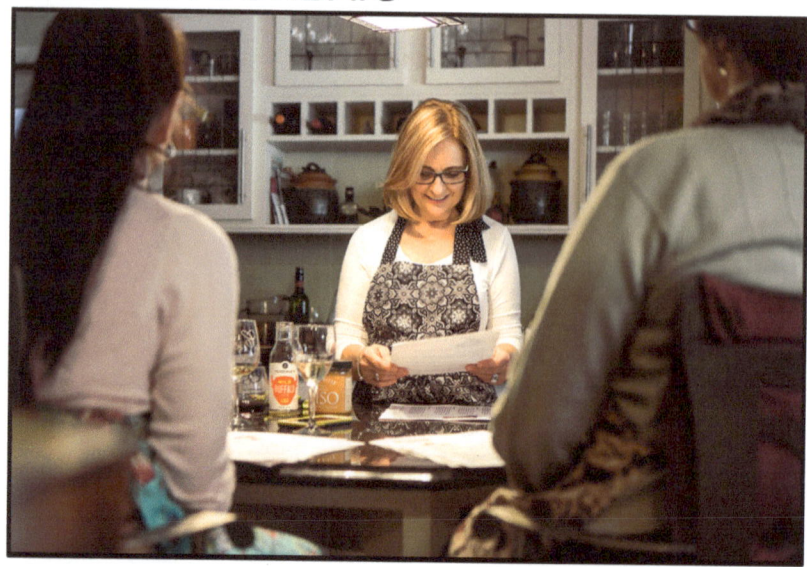

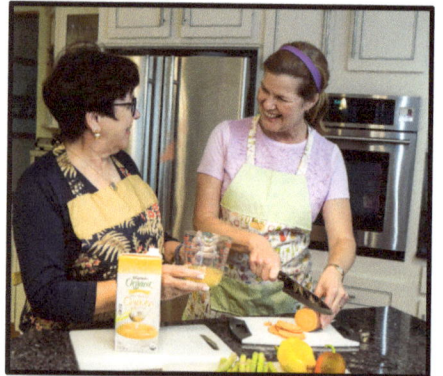

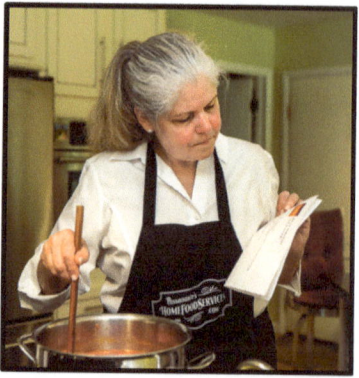

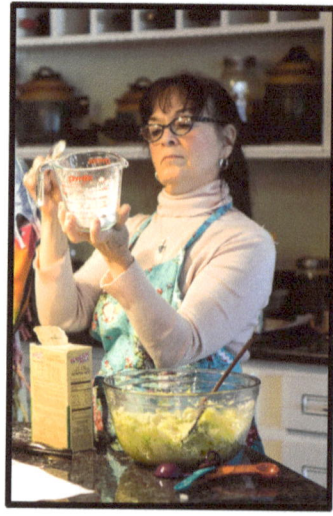

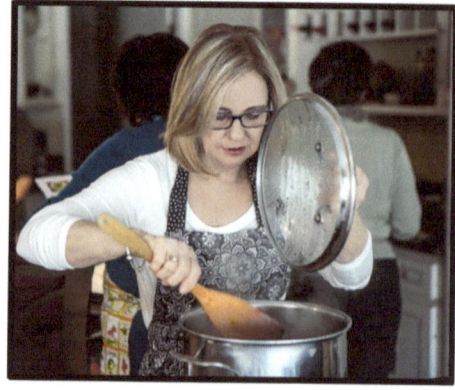

Souper Sunday classes not only educate participants on nutrition, but it's a fun afternoon filled with laughter and delicious food.

ABOUT ESSENCE INTEGRATED NUTRITION

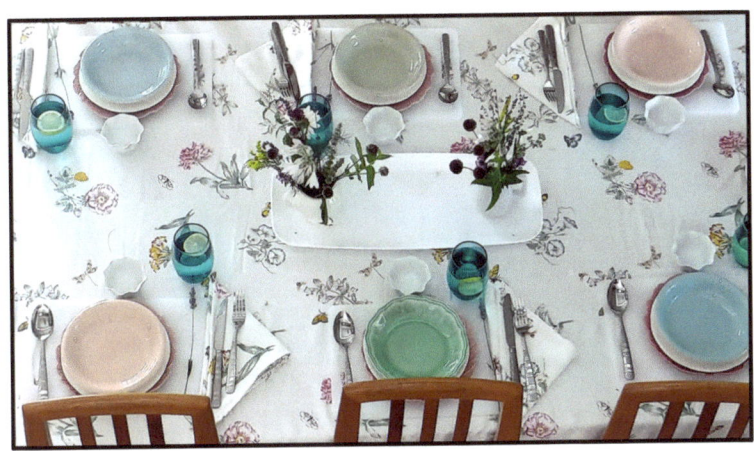

Essence Integrated Nutrition offers many options to transform your health:

ONE-ON-ONE INDIVIDUALIZED COACHING SESSIONS

Each session will leave you feeling inspired and motivated. We talk about health-related topics beyond food, seeking to bring balance to important elements of your life. I will personally and carefully guide you to make simple, attainable changes that transform your life.

GROUP COACHING SESSIONS AND CLASSES

Small group classes focus on a healthy lifestyle. Topics range from wise food choices, gut health, elimination diet protocols, detox programs, finding balance in life and more. These classes offer support and information at very affordable pricing.

COOKING CLASSES

Seasonal cooking classes are designed for a hands-on cooking experience. Each class teaches the health benefits of the food, actual preparation of the selected meal, and then a wonderful dining experience.

Essence House also offers custom designed group cooking experiences for events such as Girls' Night Out, Retirement Socials, and Wine and Dine events. I can customize an experience to meet your small group's needs.

I am also available for speaking engagements to schools and social groups on a variety of nutritional topics.

To register for a class or to customize your experience contact:
Jan Pavelco
pavelcoj@ptd.net
www.essenceintegratednutrition.com

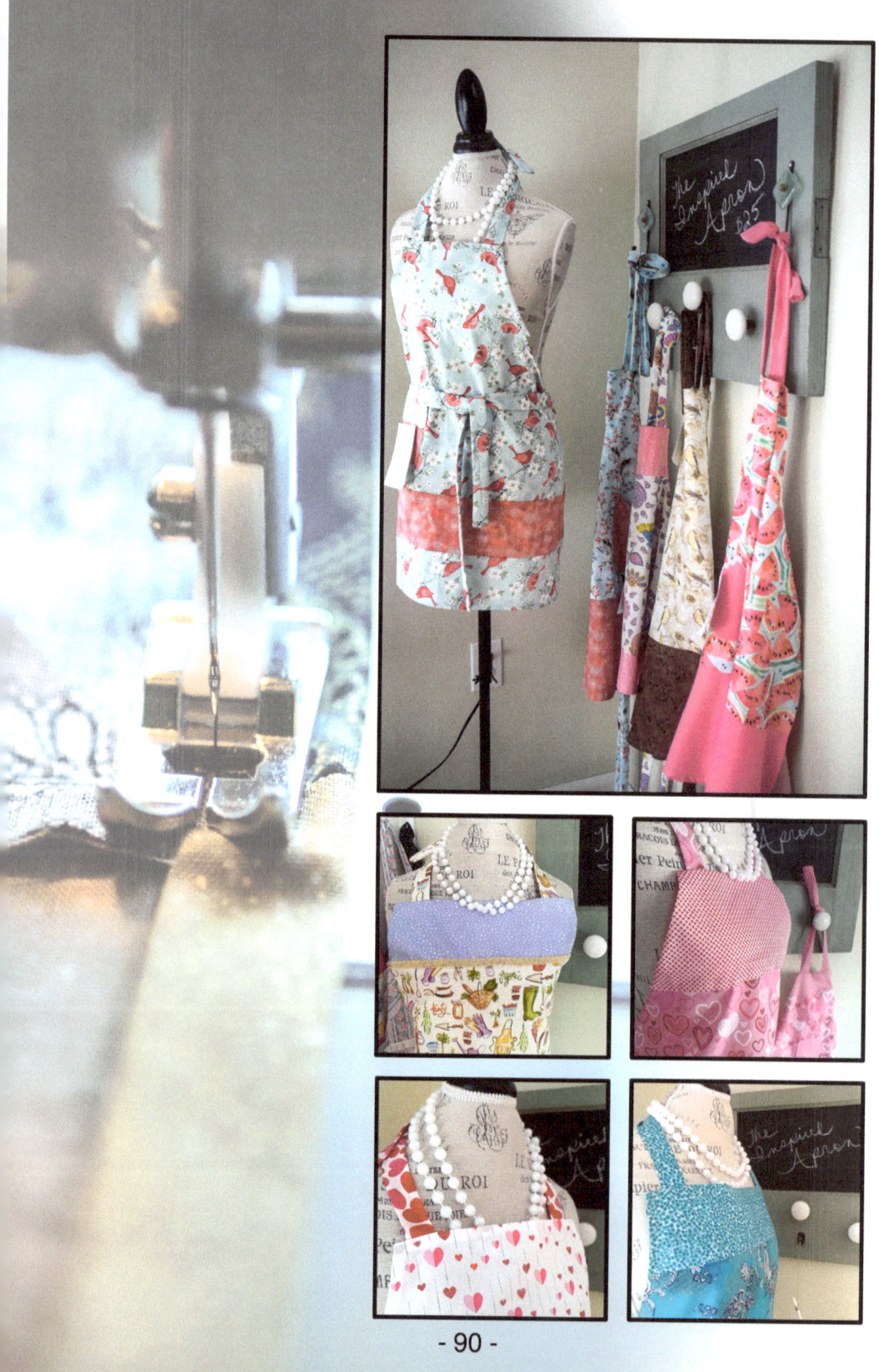

HOW TO ORDER AN INSPIRED APRON

One of my favorite creative outlets is in the making of The Inspired Apron line. To me, the simple act of putting on an apron signals the brain that you are about to do something nourishing for yourself and those you love. I wear one every single time I cook. I even started wearing them when I do the dishes. It's amazing how clean your clothes remain when you wear one.

I custom make aprons for children, women and men to order for all occasions. I ship to anywhere in the US. To place an order, you can email a request to me at pavelcoj@ptd.net. Orders are shipped within two weeks. The gift of an apron to someone is a gift from the heart.

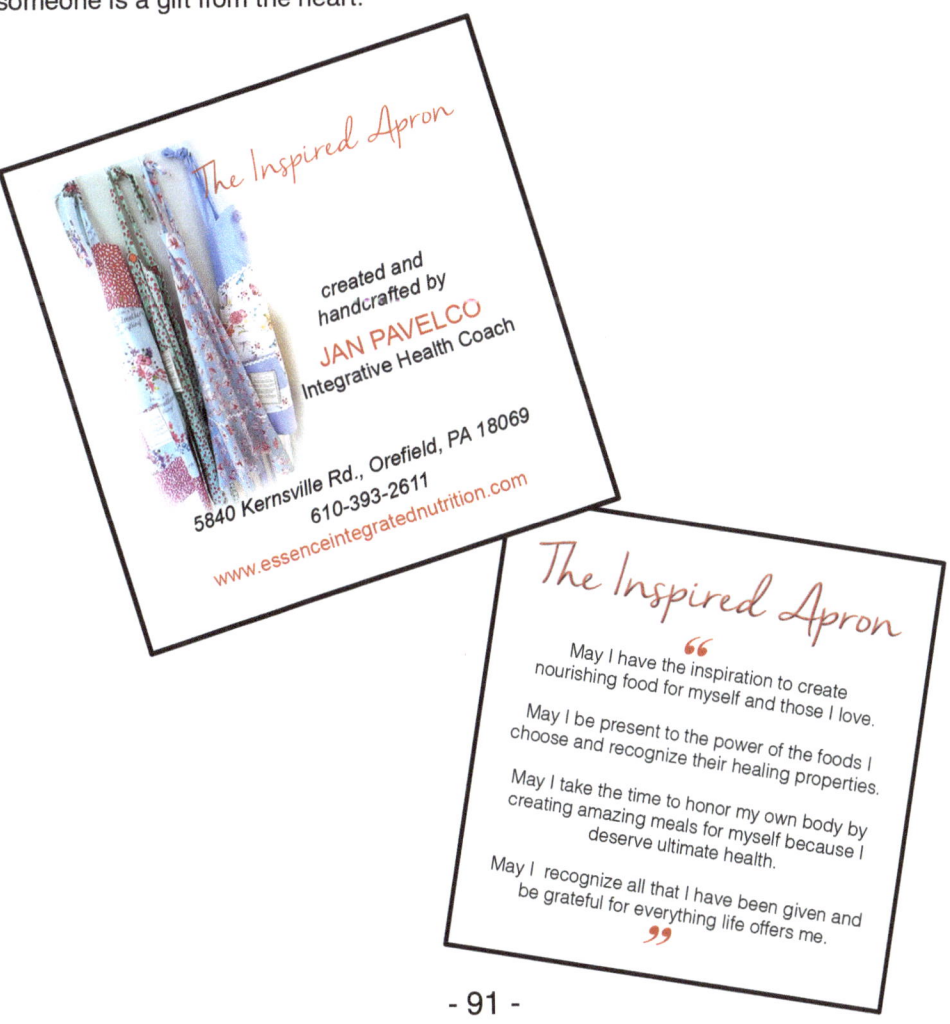

A HEARTFELT THANK YOU

Wow! It's been an unexpected journey into the heart on the road to writing this book. I thought I was going to write a simple cookbook, and then an unexpected door opened. My head and heart started to spill out all kinds of thoughts and memories. Every experience became a moment to be present to, to reflect on, and to share with the reader. All of life's experiences and studies fell into divine alignment and timing for me. This process has filled my heart with such joy. It reconnected me to my love of photography. It has made me a better person.

The road to writing this book was filled with inspiration and support from so many people at every turn. First, to my dear friend and amazingly gifted Theta healing teacher, Yolanda Perera. Over the last two and a half years that I've studied with her, there was one course called The Game of Life that really opened up all kinds of possibilities. Essence House was born, and I became a certified nutritional health coach. During this writing process, she has been a constant sounding board.

I am so grateful for the encouragement of Deborah Belaus, my long-distance bestie who told me from the start that the world didn't need another cookbook and that I had so much more to offer. Our weekly Friday phone calls provided clarity and inspiration and the subtitle of this book.

My IIN sisterhood of cheerleaders were just a Facebook message away when I wanted to share my pages with them. The trio of Michele Leitner Gootenberg, Danielle McDermott Balseiro and Beth Ledy were always just a keystroke away. Their constant words of encouragement meant more than words can express. Who knew that the seats we all chose at our conference in Miami would lead to this.

A big thank you to Marco Calderon Photography who took my portrait for the back cover and offered advice on my cover design. And to Heather Gogal Photography, another dear friend, who took her time to play with me in the kitchen to capture my picture during a soup making session. A huge thank you goes to Patrice Tritt who listened to all my concepts on our weekly rides to orchestra practice. Proofreading went easier over wine, and her heartfelt suggestions were spot on.

I want to thank each and every person who put their trust in me by attending a soup making class, bought an apron, or attended a group coaching circle. Your trust and confidence in me mean more than you can ever imagine. A special shout out to Diane, Lindsay and Cindy, my leaders of the pack and loyal supporters of each and every one of my efforts. Thank you to all of my Facebook friends who hit the like or love button on my sneak previews; and, of course, all those long-ago yearbook peeps who were indoctrinated with all those design and writing rules. Now it was my turn to use them.

Just like the academy awards, I'm sure I forgot to thank someone. What I do know is that there wasn't one person who wasn't encouraging along the way. My sisters, who always said that mom saved the best for last...thank you! Thank you Joyce Keller, Teri Hope, and Valerie Hoffman for proofing my pages. And thank you to every reader of this book. I hope these little inspirations have also opened up something in you and inspires you to live a life full of possibilities.

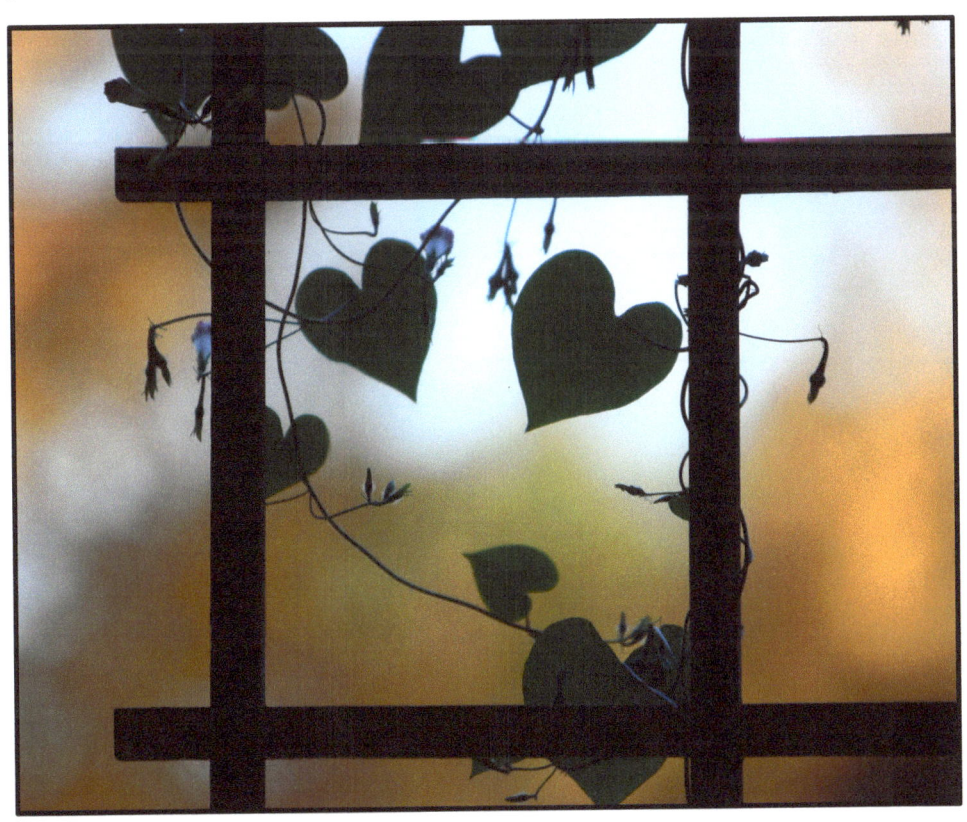

FAVORITE GEMS TO SHOP

I've listed some of my very favorite places to buy fresh, organic items. It's so very important to connect with small businesses that care about protecting the earth and offer their customers the freshest and safest products available. I encourage everyone to seek out farms and small businesses where you live and support them. They are our future!

BAD Farm, Beth and Dave Rice, 86 Weider Rd, Kempton, PA 19529

Betula's Botanica, Monica Dech, 412 Penn Avenue, West Reading, PA 19611

Crooked Row Farm, Liz Wagner, 4827 5 Point Road, New Tripoli, PA 18066. Farm stand at 3245 PA-309, Orefield, PA 18069

Eagle Point Farm, Steve and Gayle Ganser, 853 Trexlertown Road, Allentown, PA 18106

The Good Farm, John and Aimee Good, 8112 Church Rd., Germansville, PA 18053

Jersey Hollow Farm LLC, Norman & Edith Sauder, 276 Quarry Rd., Kutztown, PA 19530

Paisley and Company, Joanne Lapic, 275 W. Main Street, Kutztown, PA 19530

Red Cat Farm LLC, Teena and Michael Bailey, 6113 Memorial Rd., Germansville, PA 18053

Schocharie Ridge Apiary, Randy Spaide, 7483 Bausch Rd., New Tripoli, PA 18066

THE INSTITUTE FOR INTEGRATIVE NUTRITION

This book was inspired by my experience at the Institute for Integrative Nutrition® (IIN), where I received my training in holistic wellness and health coaching. IIN offers a truly comprehensive Health Coach Training Program that invites students to deeply explore the things that are most nourishing to them. From the physical aspects of nutrition and eating wholesome foods that work best for each individual person, to the concept of Primary Food – the idea that everything in life, including our spirituality, career, relationships, and fitness contributes to our inner and outer health – IIN helped me reach optimal health and balance.

This inner journey unleashed the passion that compels me to share what I've learned and inspire others. Beyond personal health, IIN offers training in health coaching, as well as business and marketing. Students who choose to pursue this field professionally complete the program equipped with the communication skills and branding knowledge they need to create a fulfilling career encouraging and supporting others in reaching their own health goals. From renowned wellness experts as Visiting Teachers to the convenience of their online learning platform, this school has changed my life, and I believe it will do the same for you.

I invite you to learn more about the Institute for Integrative Nutrition and explore how the Health Coach Training Program can help you transform your life. Please feel free to contact me to hear more about my personal experience with the IIN program at www.essenceintegratednutrition.com

or call IIN at (844) 315-8546 to learn more.

www.ingramcontent.com/pod-product-compliance
Lightning Source LLC
Chambersburg PA
CBHW042050290426
44110CB00001B/17